# The Easy 5-Ingredient Ketogenic Diet Cookbook

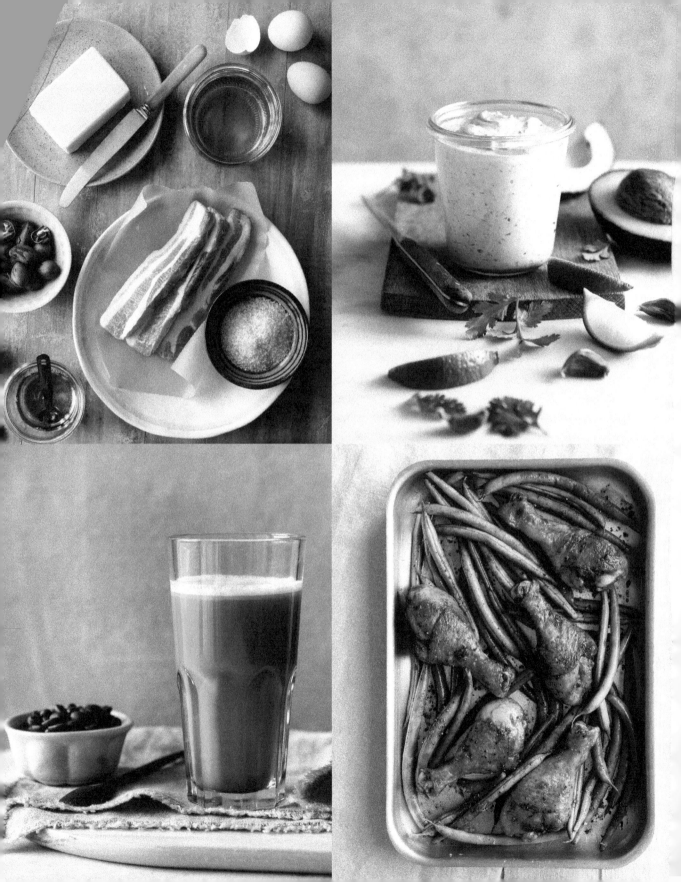

# The Easy 5-Ingredient
# KETOGENIC DIET
## Cookbook

Low-Carb, High-Fat Recipes
for Busy People on the Keto Diet

**JEN FISCH**

ROCKRIDGE
PRESS

TO MY KAIA BEAR,
MY DAUGHTER &
CHIEF TASTE TESTER

———————————————

# CONTENTS

Bulletproof Coffee, *page 19*

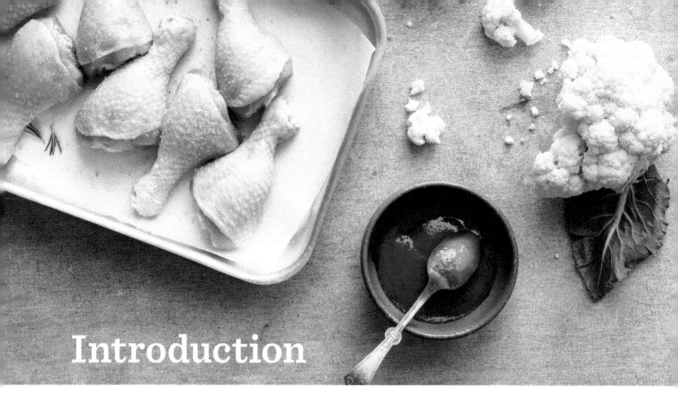

# Introduction

WHAT ON EARTH IS KETOSIS? WHAT IS A MACRO, AND HOW DO I MEASURE IT? I DECIDED TO TRY THE KETO DIET, AND I AM SO GLAD I DID.

I'm so happy you've decided to explore the ketogenic way of eating with me.

Following a keto diet has helped so many people. The keto diet is a super-low-carbohydrate diet that includes a high level of healthy fats and a moderate level of protein. My journey with low-carbohydrate eating began over a decade ago, at the recommendation of a doctor I was seeing for acupuncture. When I was 18 and 19 years old, I was diagnosed with two autoimmune disorders: psoriatic arthritis and psoriasis. I was looking for ways to alleviate pain and inflammation, and the doctor recommended

that I cut sugar out of my diet. This was the first time I had thought about the connection between food and autoimmune disorders.

I followed his advice, started on a low-carb diet, cut out sugar, and saw relief within weeks. I noticed a definite decrease in the inflammation in my joints as well as in my skin, which had been angry and red. This started me on a path of discovery, learning more about how my body reacts to various foods and finally finding an eating plan that could help me feel like my best self.

For many years I followed a mostly low-carbohydrate eating plan, but I also went through periods where I "fell off the wagon." Then, a few years ago, I started having more autoimmune issues again. My doctors thought perhaps I had Crohn's disease, but they weren't sure. After many tests and not a lot o f answers, I decided to go back to experimenting with food to see if I could help heal myself. I started by eating high-quality foods (organic, grass-fed, etc.) but with gluten-free carbs. I saw some improvement with my issues, but I just felt sluggish, and after six months of following that plan, I had gained weight thanks to those tasty gluten-free treats that are so readily available these days.

Then I came across the ketogenic diet. At first, it seemed like the induction phase to the Atkins diet, but I liked the idea of eating real foods, lower in protein, with a focus on healthy fats. I had never heard of "keto" at the time, and like many people, I felt a little confused and overwhelmed by the new keto terms. What on Earth is ketosis? What is a macro, and how do I measure it? But I decided to try the keto diet, and I am so glad I did.

Immediately I loved the challenge of creating keto-friendly meals that were quick and easy, and also delicious. I am a single mom, and I work full time. I also have an extremely busy teenage daughter, so I like to keep recipes (and everything else in my life) as simple as humanly possible. In my experience, you do not need a lot of exotic ingredients and a cupboard full of special oils to whip up amazing keto meals.

The recipes in this book will help satisfy cravings you will have for those high-carb favorites you used to eat pre-keto. Having those cravings is super normal. Most people have eaten a high-carbohydrate diet their entire lives, so it is definitely an adjustment to go keto. But I encourage you to stick with it.

My 5-ingredient recipes have made my life easier. For this book, I created as many recipes as I could that can be made in 30 minutes or less. Who has the time these days to spend hours preparing a meal? The recipes are full of flavor and healthy fats. You'll be cooking with natural, wholesome ingredients that are easy to find and that are affordable. There is no need to go to five different grocery stores just to hunt down a bunch of unfamiliar ingredients. My recipes make keto easy!

Come along with me as I guide you on your keto journey. I know you can do it. I'm excited to show you all the super-delicious ways you can make my easy, 5-ingredient, keto-friendly recipes. Let's start cooking!

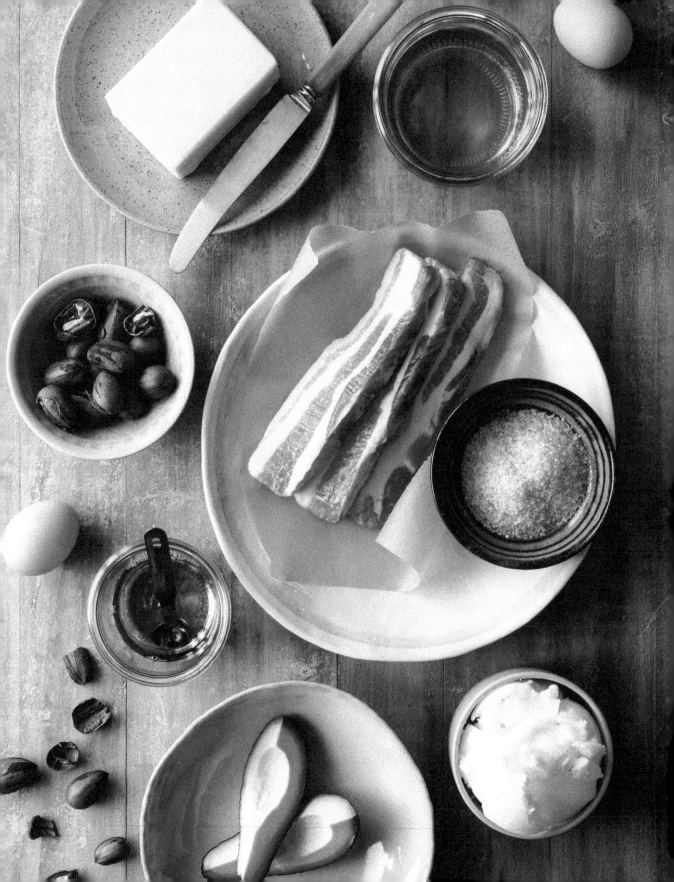

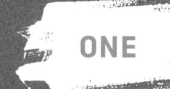

# ONE

# SIMPLE & EASY KETOGENIC COOKING

What I love most about the ketogenic lifestyle is how easy it is, both when cooking at home and eating out. The recipes in this book are simple and use familiar foods. I will show you how to turn everyday, easy-to-find ingredients into keto-friendly meals that are delicious and full of the healthy fats your body will use to fuel itself. The most important step in starting the keto diet is just starting! Don't feel intimidated: I will walk you through everything you need to know!

# HOW THE KETO DIET WORKS

Starting a new eating plan can be overwhelming. I know when I first started researching the ketogenic diet online, the materials available were confusing, and I felt like I was back in science class. But at its core, "keto" is focused on eating a diet full of healthy fats, mixed with proteins and very few carbs. Ideally, the carbs you do eat will come mainly from vegetables. Your body will switch from burning sugar and carbs for energy to burning fat/ketones for energy. This process is called "ketosis," and it puts you in the optimal state for burning body fat and losing weight. But weight loss is not the only benefit to the keto plan. Mental clarity, reduced inflammation, and increased energy are just some of the other benefits.

When you are first beginning the keto diet, you may find yourself eating more to feel full. But quickly, as you become keto-adapted, you will find that you are often not hungry at mealtime. It is important to learn to listen to your body, and if you are not hungry, you don't need to eat. I continuously remind myself of this lesson. When I am at work, I often feel like I need to eat at noon when everyone goes to lunch. However, on the weekends, without such a schedule, I can often go until 2 or 3 p.m. before eating. Allow your body to guide you, but always make sure you are drinking plenty of water and getting the proper intake of electrolytes.

The benefits of a ketogenic diet are vast, and each person has their own reason for embarking on a keto journey. For me, I was focused on reducing inflammation in my body. Removing sugar, which is extremely inflammatory, and carbohydrates has been life changing. Enabling your body to be in nutritional ketosis can be helpful for conditions such as obesity, epilepsy, neurological conditions, and more. Being a fat burner instead of a sugar burner may also boost your longevity. It seems like every week there are new studies supporting the keto lifestyle.

When starting a ketogenic diet, you may encounter new terms and have some questions:

***What is ketosis?*** Drastically restricting carbs and sugar in your diet puts your body into a state of ketosis, which is when the body burns fat (ketones) instead of glucose (carbs and sugar). When there are very few carbohydrates in the diet, the liver converts fat into fatty acids and ketone bodies. The ketone bodies pass into the brain and replace glucose as an energy source. This elevated level of ketone bodies in the blood is known as ketosis. You can often achieve a state of ketosis within the first week of starting a keto diet, which is the first step of eventually becoming keto-adapted, which can often take about a month to achieve.

***What are macros, and why are they important?*** When you first start a keto diet, you will want to calculate your "macros" and track them every day. Macros, or macronutrients, are the major nutritional elements that make up the caloric content of your food—protein, carbohydrates, fat, plus some minerals. The Centers for Disease Control and Prevention states that the typical American diet is about 50 percent carbohydrates, 15 percent protein, and 35 percent fat. In contrast, the structure of a typical keto diet is closer to 5 percent carbs, 20 to 25 percent protein, and 70 to 75 percent fat.

To find the best macros for you, you can go on Google and search for "keto macro calculator." The macro calculator will ask you to enter information (height, weight, activity level, goals, etc.), and based on that information, it will suggest your keto macros. The macros represent the upper limit of your ideal nutritional intake for each day. Macros will be broken down into calories, fat, protein, and carbohydrates. If weight loss is your goal, it is often recommended that you stay under 20 net carbs per day, which is my daily goal. I use the free Carb Manager application to track my food. You can set the preferences to net carbs.

Some people monitor their total carbohydrates while on the keto diet, and some follow net carbs; it is a personal decision. I count net carbs, which basically means that you subtract the insoluble fiber content from the total carbs because fiber is a carbohydrate that your body cannot digest. For example, ½ cup of cauliflower has 2.65 grams of carbohydrates and 1.2 grams of insoluble fiber. So you subtract the fiber from the total carbohydrates, and the net carb content of that serving is 1.45 grams.

**Is eating that much fat good for you?**
Eating 70 to 75 percent fat on the keto diet probably seems a little crazy when you are used to a typical high-carb, low-fat diet. In fact, when I first started on the keto plan, I found it easy to quit carbs but much more difficult to hit my recommended fat amount every day. The most important thing to remember is that you want to eat high-quality fats; not all fats are created equal! High-quality fats like grass-fed butter, ghee (clarified butter), grass-fed meats, organic full-fat dairy, avocados, macadamia nuts, and salmon are examples of the kinds of fats you want to consume. You should avoid low-quality fats like vegetable or canola oils. You will notice that on the keto plan, you won't be hungry as often because the high-quality fats will keep you satisfied and feeling full.

**What is intermittent fasting?** Intermittent fasting (IF) can be adopted as part of a ketogenic lifestyle. I typically eat all my food for a day within an eight-hour "eating window," which for me is typically between noon and 8 p.m. This leaves 16 hours in the day where I am intermittently fasting, but I am sleeping for a good portion of that, which makes IF pretty easy to achieve. During the IF time period, I drink Bulletproof Coffee (page 19) which is allowed on the Bulletproof Intermittent Fasting protocol, and water, but I don't consume any solid food. The Bulletproof Coffee curbs my appetite because of the fat content in the grass-fed butter and Brain Octane Oil. The longer you are on the ketogenic diet, the less hungry you will become in general, because the higher amount of fat you are eating will satiate you.

**What is keto-adapted?** Most people reach a state of ketosis within a couple of weeks of following their ketogenic macros, but becoming keto-adapted takes a little longer. Once keto-adapted, your body has switched over from using glucose as its main source of energy to using fat for energy. This process generally happens within a month of sticking to a ketogenic diet and producing a certain ketone level.

For more in-depth and scientific information on the ketogenic diet, I highly recommend everyone read *The Ketogenic Bible* by Jacob Wilson Ph.D. and Ryan Lowery. It is the most authoritative and thorough explanation of all things keto.

## GUIDELINES FOR THE KETOGENIC DIET

Switching your body from glucose burning to fat burning is a big change. And with change comes a period of adjustment. When you first begin a ketogenic diet, it is important to monitor your electrolytes, focus on nutrient-dense foods, and get plenty of rest during this time of healing for your body. Electrolytes are certain nutrients or chemicals in the body that have many important functions, including stimulating muscles, nerves, maintaining cellular function, regulating your heartbeat, and more. If your electrolytes are out of balance, you will feel tired or just "off."

**Manage your electrolytes to minimize the "keto flu" when you are first starting keto.** When you begin to follow a ketogenic diet, your body will go through a detox period as it flushes out the carbohydrates and sugar in your system. If you are like most people, you have been eating carbs your whole life, so your body will be making a big adjustment. You may experience side effects, such as lightheadedness, muscle cramps, headaches, nausea, and fatigue. Stay strong; this detox period is only temporary. The key to minimizing the side effects is managing your electrolytes in these ways:

- Drink plenty of water with electrolytes. I prefer Smartwater.
- Get plenty of salt. Consume pink Himalayan salt or broth (meat or veggie), or you can even drink shots of pickle juice.
- Eat foods rich in potassium but low in sugar, like avocado and spinach.
- Eat foods rich in magnesium, like nuts, spinach, artichokes, and fish.
- Get plenty of rest, because your body is healing.

**Drink a lot of water.** Throughout your keto journey, you will need to drink a lot of water, likely more than you are currently drinking. In the beginning stages of the diet, you will be shedding a lot of water. The carbs in your body tend to hold on to water, and when you stop eating them, your body will begin to release that water, so you need

# Ketogenic or Paleo?

## KETO AND PALEO ARE TWO DIFFERENT EATING PLANS, BUT THE TERMS OFTEN GET USED INTERCHANGEABLY.

*A TYPICAL PALEO DIET* is not as high in fat or as low in carbs as the keto diet is. Paleo is all about eating like people did several thousand years ago, when there were no processed foods and they consumed foods they could hunt, like meats, and gather, like nuts, seeds, and plants. On a Paleo diet you can eat sweet potatoes and other high-carbohydrate vegetables like carrots. There are many types of Paleo diets, but on a standard Paleo diet, the macros tend to be closer to 20 percent carbs, 15 percent protein, and 65 percent fat.

*ON THE KETO DIET*, you shouldn't eat those high-carb vegetables and starches because they will raise your glucose levels and kick you out of ketosis. Keto macros are 5 percent carbs, 20 percent protein, and 75 percent fat. To successfully follow a ketogenic diet, your body must be in a state of ketosis; otherwise, you are simply following a low-carb eating plan.

*DAIRY IS ANOTHER DIFFERENTIATOR.* On keto, full-fat dairy can be a great way to help you get your healthy fats, but you don't have to eat dairy. In the most traditional form of Paleo diet, dairy is avoided completely, but now there are many types of Paleo plans, and some do allow dairy products.

*IT IS POSSIBLE TO FOLLOW THE KETO DIET WHILE ALSO FOLLOWING SOME PALEO PRINCIPLES*, particularly a focus on natural, high-quality foods. I always recommend that whenever you can, you use the highest-quality ingredients you can afford. In addition, you can swap out certain ingredients for more Paleo-friendly ingredients; for example, you can replace butter with ghee, and heavy whipping cream with coconut milk.

to replenish it. A good guide is to make sure you get *at least* half your body weight in ounces of water daily. For example, if you weigh 200 pounds, you should drink at least 100 ounces of water (a bit more than 3 quarts) every day.

***Get plenty of salt.*** In a standard American diet, people are typically eating foods that have a lot of salt added to them: bread, for example. On keto you are not, so don't be afraid to salt your food (using high-quality salt), and if you feel like you still need more salt, sip some meat or vegetable broth. I recommend pink Himalayan salt because it has more minerals than traditional table salt, such as potassium, magnesium, copper, and iron.

***Find easy ways to get your fat in.*** It may sound daunting to consume 70 to 75 percent of your daily diet in fat, but there are lots of easy ways to take it in throughout the day. The easiest way is to add butter and/or healthy oils to almost everything you eat.

***Do your research before eating out.*** One of the things I really love about the keto diet is that I can find something keto-friendly on almost any restaurant menu, but it does take some practice! If you can, before you go out, look online at the restaurant's menu to figure out the good keto options. Meat and vegetables are usually a great place to start. Be careful with sauces, dressings, and marinades; they can have lots of hidden carbohydrates. When in doubt, ask your server for the ingredients in the sauces, and if they don't know, I suggest asking to have the sauce left off. Restaurants are used to special requests, so don't be afraid to ask for exactly what you do and don't want.

## KITCHEN EQUIPMENT

You don't need to have a bunch of fancy equipment in your kitchen to cook the recipes in this book. But you should have a few key items for everyday use.

### MUST HAVE

***Measuring cups and measuring spoons*** You will want to make sure you are measuring items accurately rather than just eyeballing them, especially for the baking recipes. And if weight loss is your goal, portion sizes will be important, too.

***Spatula, slotted spoon, large spoon, whisk, tongs, and rubber scraper*** I tend to buy cute rubber scrapers all the time, but you really only need one of each of these six tools.

***Cutting board*** Ideally you should have two: one for vegetables and one for meat.

***Knives*** Buy one or two quality chef's knives. A quality paring knife and a 6-inch chef's knife are a good start. I bought mine on sale at Williams-Sonoma.

***Cheese grater/zester*** It is less expensive to grate your own cheese than to buy it preshredded. Some graters even have storage containers attached to them for convenience. A citrus zester can also be handy if you find a cheese grater to be too large. In a few of these recipes, we'll also be zesting/shredding citrus and vegetables.

**Baking sheet**  You will want to have one large baking sheet for one-pan meals and for baking.

**9-by-13-inch baking pan**  I like to use a deeper baking pan for roasting vegetables and meat. I also use it for my egg frittatas. The one I use all the time is an easy-to-clean Le Creuset enameled cast iron pan.

**9-by-5-inch loaf pan**  This is a standard-size loaf pan that I use for baking my Keto Bread (page 78).

**Muffin tin**  You'll need a standard muffin tin for several of these recipes. I use a jumbo muffin tin for my BLTA Cups (page 115), but a standard tin will work here, too.

**8-inch glass baking dish**  A smaller deep glass pan is great for baking desserts or making foods in smaller portions.

**10- or 12-inch skillet**  I like to use a non-stick skillet because they are easy to clean and work really well for keto staples like eggs. Professional chefs would say a nonstick pan won't achieve the same level of sear as a stainless skillet, but for my purposes it works just fine. If you prefer a stainless skillet, you will just need to put a bit more elbow grease into the cleaning process. Whichever you choose, buy one with a lid.

**Saucepans**  Having a small (2-quart) and a large (4.5-quart) saucepan will allow you to make most recipes.

**Slow cooker**  A slow cooker, like the original Crock-Pot and other brands, is very handy for making easy one-dish meals,

especially in the winter. I love letting my house fill up with delicious aromas as the food cooks all day long. The cooker I have is super simple—it doesn't have a timer or any other fancy mechanisms—and it works like a dream. I use a 6-quart slow cooker for all the slow cooker recipes in this book.

**Colander**  A colander is important for washing fresh fruits and vegetables. Just a medium-size colander should be adequate unless you are cooking for a crowd.

**Mixing bowls**  A set of nesting mixing bowls is very helpful when making a recipe. I have a set that I have had for at least 10 years, and I use the pieces all the time.

**Ice pop molds**  There are a lot of fun ice pop molds out there, and you can choose any shape to make delicious keto-friendly ice pops.

**Parchment paper**  I use parchment paper for everything from egg frittatas to roasting vegetables to making cheese chips. I buy the precut squares. It says on the box that parchment paper can be used for temperatures up to 425°F. (I learned the hard way!)

**You will also need either a blender or a food processor:**

**Blender**  A blender is a great tool for making smoothies, coffee drinks, soups, and sauces. If you don't have a blender, you can get away with doing what I do, which is use my food processor for everything!

# FOODS TO ENJOY
## HIGH FAT / LOW CARB (BASED ON NET CARBS)

### MEATS & SEAFOOD

Beef (ground beef, steak, etc.)

Chicken

Crab

Crawfish

Duck

Fish

Goose

Lamb

Lobster

Mussels

Octopus

Pork (pork chops, bacon, etc.)

Quail

Sausage (without fillers)

Scallops

Shrimp

Veal

Venison

### DAIRY

Blue cheese dressing

Burrata cheese

Cottage cheese

Cream cheese

Eggs

Greek yogurt (full-fat)

Grilling cheese

Halloumi cheese

Heavy (whipping) cream

Homemade whipped cream

Kefalotyri cheese

Mozzarella cheese

Provolone cheese

Queso blanco

Ranch dressing

Ricotta cheese

Unsweetened almond milk

Unsweetened coconut milk

### NUTS & SEEDS

Almonds

Brazil nuts

Chia seeds

Flaxseeds

Hazelnuts

Macadamia nuts

Peanuts (in moderation)

Pecans

Pine nuts

Pumpkin seeds

Sacha inchi seeds

Sesame seeds

Walnuts

### FRUITS & VEGETABLES

Alfalfa sprouts

Asparagus

Avocados

Bell peppers

Blackberries

Blueberries

Broccoli

Cabbage

Carrots (in moderation)

Cauliflower

Celery

Chicory

Coconut

Cranberries

Cucumbers

Garlic (in moderation)

Green beans

Herbs

Jicama

Lemons

Limes

Mushrooms

Okra

Olives

Onions (in moderation)

Pickles

Pumpkin

Radishes

Raspberries

Salad greens

Scallions

Spaghetti squash (in moderation)

Strawberries

Tomatoes (in moderation)

Zucchini

# FOODS TO AVOID

## LOW FAT / HIGH CARB (BASED ON NET CARBS)

### MEATS & MEAT ALTERNATIVES

Deli meat (some, not all)
Hot dogs (with fillers)
Sausage (with fillers)
Seitan
Tofu

### DAIRY

Almond milk (sweetened)
Coconut milk (sweetened)
Milk
Soy milk (regular)
Yogurt (regular)

### NUTS & SEEDS

Cashews
Chestnuts
Pistachios

### FRUITS & VEGETABLES

Apples
Apricots
Artichokes
Bananas
Beans (all varieties)
Boysenberries
Burdock root
Butternut squash
Cantaloupe
Cherries
Chickpeas
Corn
Currants
Dates
Edamame
Eggplant
Elderberries
Gooseberries
Grapes
Honeydew melon
Huckleberries
Kiwifruits
Leeks
Mangos
Oranges
Parsnips
Peaches
Peas
Pineapples
Plantains
Plums
Potatoes
Prunes
Raisins
Sweet potatoes
Taro root
Turnips
Water chestnuts
Winter squash
Yams

**Food processor** I use my food processor a lot for making these recipes. I have a small one, the Cuisinart Mini-Prep, because there are only two people in my household. It costs about $40, and I use it all the time.

## NICE TO HAVE

**Mixer** I use an electric hand mixer I've had for years, but if you have a countertop mixer, that is an awesome tool. A mixer is particularly helpful for making desserts. If you don't have either, you can also use a whisk and get a great arm workout at the same time.

**Kitchen scale** I do not have a kitchen scale, but I know it is a key item for many people who are trying to lose weight on keto. They use it to measure portions, especially for meat and other proteins.

**Immersion blender** This tool is very handy for quickly blending soups and sauces right in the pan or bowl, instead of in a food processor or countertop blender.

**Rolling pin** If you have a rolling pin, it will come in handy for making dishes like pinwheels. If you don't have one, I have also used a wine bottle and it worked just fine!

**Basting brush** I like using a basting brush with olive oil so that you don't dump too much, but if you don't have one, you can also use a leafy green or paper towel instead.

**Cooling rack** For several of these recipes, I transfer a finished dish from the oven to a cooling rack. If you don't have one, setting your hot dishes on trivets or pot holders will work, too.

# KETO PANTRY ESSENTIALS

It is wise to have a well-stocked pantry when you are cooking keto meals. You do not need any exotic cooking ingredients; you just need to have the basics. Each recipe in this book has only 5 main ingredients, but the following 5 basic cooking staples do *not* count toward those ingredients.

## KETO COOKING STAPLES

1. Pink Himalayan salt
2. Freshly ground black pepper
3. Ghee (clarified butter, without dairy; buy grass-fed if you can)
4. Olive oil
5. Grass-fed butter

In addition to these 5 staples, there are 10 key perishable ingredients you will want to always have on hand. I recommend that you purchase organic/all-natural whenever possible.

## KETO PERISHABLES

1. Eggs (pasture-raised, if you can)
2. Avocados
3. Bacon (uncured)
4. Cream cheese (full-fat; or use a dairy-free alternative)
5. Sour cream (full-fat; or use a dairy-free alternative)
6. Heavy whipping cream or coconut milk (full-fat; I buy the coconut milk in a can)

7. Garlic (fresh or pre-minced in a jar)
8. Cauliflower
9. Meat (grass-fed, if you can)
10. Greens (spinach, kale, or arugula)

In addition, the following are some of my favorite products that I always keep in my kitchen. Some are staples and some are snacks or sweet treats. In the Resources section, I tell you where to find these products. I even have discount codes you can use for some of them!

## FAVORITE KETO PRODUCTS

***Vital Farms Pasture-Raised Eggs*** The first thing that attracted me to this brand of eggs was their beautiful packaging and the fact that these eggs are pasture raised. The yolks are orange, and the eggs are delicious; buying pasture-raised eggs definitely makes a difference. Fresh pasture-raised eggs are even better if you have a local farmers' market.

***Kerrygold Butter*** Grass-fed butter just tastes better; once you switch, you will never go back. Kerrygold, from Ireland, has a higher fat content. There are other grass-fed brands, but Kerrygold is widely available at Whole Foods, Costco, Trader Joe's, Walmart, and Safeway. It comes unsalted and salted; I use salted for almost everything.

***Bulletproof Brain Octane Oil*** Bulletproof is a brand that makes a variety of high-quality keto products. My favorites are their coffee, ghee, and Brain Octane Oil. The Brain Octane Oil is one of my keto secret weapons because it is a very easy way to add high-quality fats to anything you eat. One tablespoon of the oil has 14 grams of fat, no flavor, and no smell. I use Brain Octane Oil in my Bulletproof Coffee, often called "butter coffee," and there are many other ways to use it.

***Bulletproof Ghee*** I trust the quality of Bulletproof products, so I also purchase their ghee. Ghee is clarified butter (with no dairy), which has a high smoke point, so it is great to use for cooking. Just like with butter, I recommend grass-fed ghee. A good percentage of people who do the keto diet do it dairy-free, so ghee is a perfect replacement for butter in cooking, as well as a tasty addition to Bulletproof Coffee.

***Primal Palate Spice Mixes*** Seasoning can really enhance a dish and a meal. I have fallen in love with the seasoning mixes from Primal Palate. Their spices are the highest quality available, and they make amazing spice blends, like Breakfast Blend, Super Gyro, and Garam Masala, which will take your dishes to a new level.

***Perfect Keto MCT Oil Powder*** This product is wonderful for adding high-quality fats in dishes and drinks. Oils can be messy and of course add an oily texture to drinks. MCT oil powder adds fats, and it has a nice creamy texture that works perfectly in beverages like coffee or smoothies. I also use it in baking because it doesn't have a taste, and it just adds healthy fats.

**Perfect Keto Protein Collagen MCT Oil Powder** Also by Perfect Keto, this dairy-free protein powder has collagen in it, which I love. The production of collagen in our bodies slows down as we age, so consuming products like this one with added collagen can help combat some of the collagen loss. Collagen is beneficial for the joints, hair, and nails, among other things.

**Fat Snax Cookies** These healthy, fat-packed cookies come in delicious flavors and are Paleo-friendly, keto-friendly, and organic. My daughter loves to make keto-friendly ice cream sandwiches with them.

**Keto Kookies** Another sweet cookie option, Keto Kookie was created by two friends who lost weight on a ketogenic diet and decided to launch their own brand. They come in delicious flavors, and the texture is moist and chewy.

**Trader Joe's Rosemary Marcona Almonds** I am obsessed with these nuts. If you have never had a Marcona almond, they are an oilier almond with a flatter shape and a delicate taste. Trader Joe's sells a couple of varieties, but rosemary is my favorite.

**Miracle Noodles and Miracle Rice** These two products really expand what you can do with keto cooking. Miracle Noodles and Miracle Rice are gluten-free, soy-free, and calorie-free and have zero net carbs. They have a variety of noodle styles so you can make all your favorite noodle dishes in a keto-friendly way.

**Primal Kitchen Products** For mayo and salad dressings, I love Primal Kitchen's products. If you aren't going to make your own, this is the brand I would trust. Their mayo is made with avocado oil and is sugar-free.

I'm also fond of using the following general, non-keto-specific products for my recipes. They taste great, fulfill my dietary requirements, and tend to be reasonably priced. All of my recipes were tested and developed using these products, but feel free to substitute alternatives if you have your own favorites!

- Annie's Organic Honey Mustard Dressing
- Boar's Head or Citterio Pancetta
- Bob's Red Mill Coconut Flour
- Elvio's Chimichurri Sauce
- Frank's RedHot Sauce
- Justin's All Natural Peanut Butter
- Kettle & Fire Bone Broth
- Lily's Sugar-Free Chocolate Chips
- Mission Low-Carb Whole-Wheat Tortillas
- Muir Glen Organic Diced Tomatoes with Italian Seasoning
- Organic Girl Fresh Salad Greens: Baby Spinach, Baby Kale, Romaine Hearts, Romaine Leaves, Butter Lettuce, Red Romaine, Baby Arugula
- Primal Kitchen sauces and salad dressings: Mayonnaise, Greek Vinaigrette, Caesar with Avocado Oil, Ranch
- Rao's Homemade Tomato Sauce
- Spicy Red Pepper Miso Mayo

- Swerve Natural Sweetener
- Trader Joe's Almond Flour
- Trader Joe's Chunky Blue Cheese Dressing
- Trader Joe's Coconut Oil Cooking Spray
- Trader Joe's Frozen Medium Cooked Shrimp
- Trader Joe's Organic Chia Seeds
- Trader Joe's Organic Coconut Cream
- Trader Joe's Organic Full-Fat Unsweetened Coconut Milk (13.5-ounce can); it tends to separate, so stir after opening and before measuring
- Trader Joe's Sliced Prosciutto
- Wild Planet Alaska Wild Canned Salmon
- Zevia All-Natural Root Beer

# KETO COOKING

The ketogenic diet can seem complicated at first, but it is really about simplifying your eating habits. I am successful when I eat simple meals made with high-quality, natural ingredients. The recipes in this book are good examples of this simple approach, because they each have just 5 main ingredients. By planning your shopping trips around these recipes, you will be able to set yourself up for success. In my experience, the better your plan, the more successful you will be on your keto diet. A "plan" can be different for everyone. For example, I always pack keto-friendly snacks when I go out of town and when I have all-day meetings. Otherwise, it is easy to give in to what is available. For others, preparing an entire week's worth of food on the weekend may be the best plan for success.

***Use the highest-quality ingredients you can afford.*** Processed and lower-quality foods can cause inflammation in your body, which is what a ketogenic diet is fighting against. So do what you can to keep your diet as clean as possible with real, high-quality foods.

***Remove non-keto foods from your home.*** Give away your carb-filled pantry items to your friends, neighbors, coworkers, or a charity. Just get them out of the house to set yourself up for success.

***Keep your food as simple as possible.*** Stick to recipes like the ones in this book that use real food and do not have lots of ingredients. Keto is made to be simple.

***Track your food throughout the day.*** Get in the habit of entering your meals into an app like Carb Manager. Not every meal has to add up to perfect keto macros, but the more mindful you are throughout the day, the easier it will be to reach your goals. The macro goals you are aiming for every day are in fat, protein, carbs, and calories.

***Plan your meals.*** Prepping meals ahead of time so you always have food on hand is the key to success for many people. Make sure your refrigerator and pantry are stocked with staples so that when those cravings hit, you can satisfy them with an appropriate low-carb, high-fat option.

***Prep and store ingredients ahead of time.*** Hardboiled eggs make perfect last-minute snacks that you can prepare ahead of time and have ready in the refrigerator. I also like to prepare small zip-top bags of veggies, nuts, slices of cheese, and other keto-friendly snacks, and keep them available in the fridge for grab and go. Also, you will find that rinsing and cutting up vegetables you plan to use for the next week's recipes is a helpful way to cut down on your evening meal-prep time.

***Cook in bulk.*** It is usually cheaper to buy meat and poultry in larger quantities, so don't be reluctant to cook a week's worth at one time and store it in the refrigerator and freezer. It will save you a lot of time throughout the week.

***Don't be afraid of new food combinations.*** The ketogenic diet gives you the opportunity to get creative with delicious high-fat ingredients you may not be very familiar with.

***Don't be afraid of salt and seasoning.*** You can give a dish as simple as eggs a totally different taste profile simply by using different seasonings. Have fun with flavors.

***Commit.*** It takes about a month to become fully keto-adapted, which is when your body has fully switched over and has become super-efficient at using fat/ketones as fuel. Keto is meant to be a long-term way of eating, so give your body time to heal and adjust.

# About the Recipes

**IN THIS BOOK YOU WILL FIND 130 EASY, 5-INGREDIENT RECIPES FOR EVERY MEAL.**

Over half the recipes take less than 30 minutes to prepare, and whenever possible I tried to minimize the pots and pans needed because I love for cleanup to be easy, too.

The recipes in this book have helpful labels you can look for:

*ONE POT* These recipes can be made in a single pot or bowl.

*ONE PAN* These recipes can be made in a single skillet, baking dish, or other cooking vessel.

*30-MINUTE* These recipes will take 30 minutes or less for prep and cooking.

*NO COOK* These recipes do not involve any cooking.

*VEGETARIAN* These recipes do not contain any meat.

Each recipe in the book calls for just 5 main ingredients and uses some of the 5 pantry ingredients as well: pink Himalayan salt, freshly ground black pepper, grass-fed ghee, olive oil, and grass-fed butter. You'll find the nutritional information as well as the macro breakdowns (see page 3) at the bottom of each recipe.

Every recipe also includes at least one tip:

*SUBSTITUTION TIP* This tip makes suggestions for replacing or swapping out ingredients.

*INGREDIENT TIP* This tip recommends easy or alternative ways of prepping ingredients.

*VARIATIONS* This tip suggests other flavor or ingredient combinations you can use in the basic dish to easily change a recipe.

Most of the recipes in the book are made for two people, because I originally created my recipes for me and my daughter. And through my followers, I've discovered that a two-person recipe yield is very popular. If you're expecting more people, just multiply the ingredients.

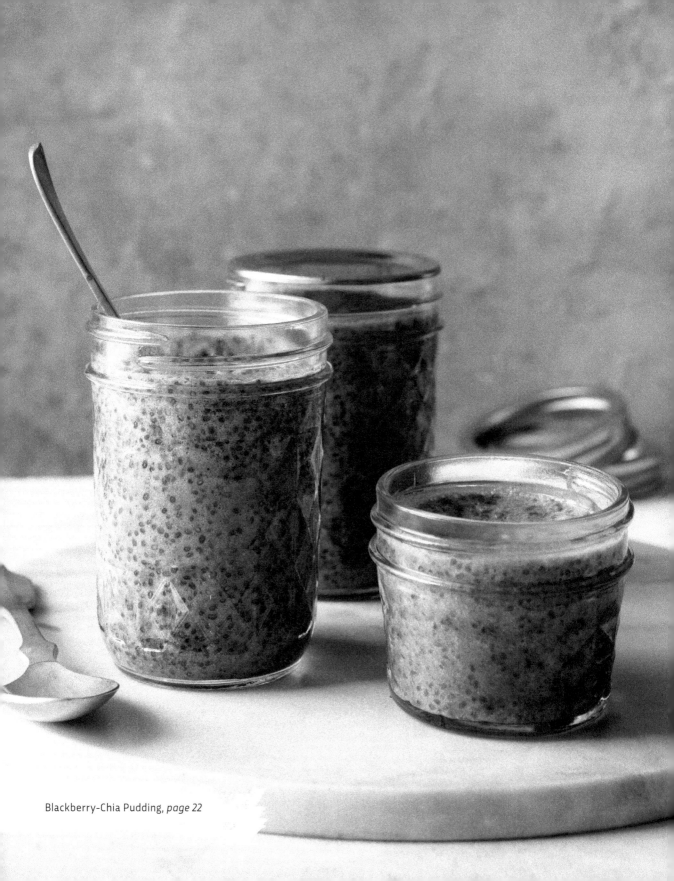

Blackberry-Chia Pudding, *page 22*

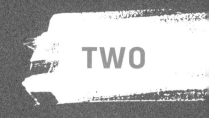

# TWO

# SMOOTHIES & BREAKFASTS

The ketogenic diet and breakfast foods are a perfect pair. For just one ingredient, eggs, there are endless ways you can get creative. The recipes in this chapter are some of the favorites I often make for my daughter and me. During the busy work and school week, I generally stick to Bulletproof Coffee or an Americano with heavy whipping cream for breakfast. But on the weekends, I love to make large keto breakfasts. These breakfast recipes will show you how you can take some of your favorite morning dishes, such as sugar- and carb-filled smoothies and pancakes, and turn them into easy, keto-friendly options.

# BULLETPROOF COFFEE

Bulletproof Coffee is a staple beverage in a lot of keto diets. I love it and honestly feel like Wonder Woman after I drink a cup. One of the biggest benefits for me is being able to extend my Bulletproof intermittent fast because the fat-filled coffee keeps me satiated until lunchtime. If you are not using Bulletproof Coffee for fasting and instead would like to add protein or collagen, you can do that as well.

**30-MINUTE**
**ONE PAN**
**NO COOK**

**SERVES 1**
**PREP** 5 minutes

1½ cups hot coffee

2 tablespoons MCT oil powder or Bulletproof Brain Octane Oil

2 tablespoons butter or ghee

**Per Serving**
Calories: 463; Total Fat: 51g; Carbs: 0g; Net Carbs: 0g; Fiber: 0g; Protein: 1g

1. Pour the hot coffee into the blender.

2. Add the oil powder and butter, and blend until thoroughly mixed and frothy.

3. Pour into a large mug and enjoy.

**VARIATIONS**

If you want to add protein to your Bulletproof Coffee, here are a couple of suggestions. If you are intermittent fasting, you don't want to add protein because it will end your fast. If you aren't fasting, then try these easy ways to create a more filling breakfast drink:

- Raw egg: To add protein, replace the MCT oil powder with 1 raw egg. Sounds weird, I know, but the egg adds an appealing creamy texture, and although the hot coffee cooks the egg, I promise there will be no hint of cooked proteins.
- Protein and collagen powder: You could also add a scoop or two of protein powder. I like Perfect Keto Collagen, which has a great chocolate flavor that is especially tasty in coffee. The Keto Collagen Powder contains grass-fed collagen, MCT oil powder, and protein powder. The collagen is a good anti-inflammatory addition.
- Spiced: Add 1 teaspoon of cinnamon and a little sweetener to your Bulletproof mixture for a delicious spiced version.

*INGREDIENT TIP* If you're new to the keto diet, you will want to start slow with the Brain Octane Oil. It is powerful, so you'll want to work your way up to 2 tablespoons over the course of a few weeks.

# BERRY-AVOCADO SMOOTHIE

This smoothie is my favorite. It's so delicious, and it's filled with healthy fat, potassium, magnesium, and fiber. Use the liquid stevia if you prefer sweeter smoothies.

30-MINUTE
ONE PAN
NO COOK
VEGETARIAN

**SERVES 2**
**PREP** 5 minutes

1 cup unsweetened full-fat coconut milk

1 scoop Perfect Keto Exogenous Ketone Powder in peaches and cream

½ avocado

1 cup fresh spinach

½ cup berries, fresh or frozen (no sugar added if frozen)

½ cup ice cubes

¼ teaspoon liquid stevia (optional)

**Per Batch**
Calories: 709; Total Fat: 68g; Carbs: 27g; Net Carbs: 14g; Fiber: 12g; Protein: 8g

**Per Serving**
Calories: 355; Total Fat: 40g; Carbs: 16g; Net Carbs: 8g; Fiber: 6g; Protein: 4g

1. In a blender, combine the coconut milk, protein powder, avocado, spinach, berries, ice, and stevia (if using).

2. Blend until thoroughly mixed and frothy.

3. Pour into two glasses and enjoy.

*INGREDIENT TIP* Adding avocado to a smoothie recipe may sound unusual, but it adds nutrition and healthy fat and contributes a creamy smoothness.

# ALMOND BUTTER SMOOTHIE

My daughter feels like she is drinking a milkshake when I make this smoothie for her, but it is very healthy. I love knowing that I can give her something delicious that is also powering her body and mind for hours and hours. Add the liquid stevia, a natural sweetener, if you prefer sweeter smoothies.

30-MINUTE
ONE PAN
NO COOK
VEGETARIAN

**SERVES 2**
**PREP** 5 minutes

1 cup unsweetened full-fat coconut milk

1 scoop Perfect Keto Exogenous Ketone Powder in chocolate sea salt

½ avocado

2 tablespoons almond butter

½ cup berries, fresh or frozen (no sugar added if frozen)

½ cup ice cubes

¼ teaspoon liquid stevia (optional)

**Per Batch**
Calories: 892; Total Fat: 85g; Carbs: 31g; Net Carbs: 17g; Fiber: 14g; Protein: 14g

**Per Serving**
Calories: 446; Total Fat: 43g; Carbs: 16g; Net Carbs: 9g; Fiber: 7g; Protein: 7g

1. In a blender, combine the coconut milk, protein powder, avocado, almond butter, berries, ice, and stevia (if using).

2. Blend until thoroughly mixed and frothy.

3. Pour into two glasses and enjoy.

*INGREDIENT TIP* You can add 1 teaspoon of turmeric powder to boost this smoothie's anti-inflammatory power. Or you can add 1 tablespoon of chia seeds that have been soaked in coconut milk for at least 20 minutes. The seeds will add extra fiber, iron, calcium, and omega-3 fatty acids to the smoothie.

# BLACKBERRY-CHIA PUDDING

I developed this recipe one day when I had a can of coconut milk in my pantry and wanted to find a new way to use it. I reached out to my lovely Instagram followers, and someone suggested I make chia pudding. I whipped up the pudding using blackberries, which are a great low-carb option and they add a lot of great flavor and texture. This sweet treat could be a dessert, but I also enjoy it as a super-delicious breakfast. Loaded with fiber, iron, calcium, and omega-3 fatty acids, chia seeds are one of the most nutritious foods on the planet. It's puzzling that such a tiny food can have so many health benefits, right? The chia seeds soak in the coconut milk and soften overnight to help set the pudding mixture. Chia seeds help slow digestion, and the fat content of this dish helps keep you feeling satisfied for hours.

ONE PAN
NO COOK
VEGETARIAN

**SERVES 2**
**PREP** 10 minutes, plus overnight to set

1 cup unsweetened full-fat coconut milk

1 teaspoon liquid stevia

1 teaspoon vanilla extract

½ cup blackberries, fresh or frozen (no sugar added if frozen)

¼ cup chia seeds

**Per Batch**
Calories: 873; Total Fat: 75g; Carbs: 46g; Net Carbs: 15g; Fiber: 30g; Protein: 15g

**Per Serving**
Calories: 437; Total Fat: 38g; Carbs: 23g; Net Carbs: 8g; Fiber: 15g; Protein: 8g

1. In a food processor (or blender), process the coconut milk, stevia, and vanilla until the mixture starts to thicken.

2. Add the blackberries, and process until thoroughly mixed and purple. Fold in the chia seeds.

3. Divide the mixture between two small cups with lids, and refrigerate overnight or up to 3 days before serving.

*COOKING TIP* The first time I made this recipe, I tried whisking the mixture by hand in a bowl instead of using a food processor or blender, assuming it would thicken overnight, but it did not. So using a food processor or blender is a must.

# DOUBLE-PORK FRITTATA

I love a frittata. I used to always make them with cheese, but one day I was out of cheese and decided to just add heavy whipping cream. The recipe ended up so fluffy and delicious that I have never gone back. For this recipe, I use all-natural pork lard, available from Fatworks as well as most butchers, or you can use the lard from bacon.

**30-MINUTE**

**SERVES 4**
**PREP** 5 minutes
**COOK** 25 minutes

1 tablespoon butter or pork lard

8 large eggs

1 cup heavy (whipping) cream

Pink Himalayan salt

Freshly ground black pepper

4 ounces pancetta, chopped

2 ounces prosciutto, thinly sliced

1 tablespoon chopped fresh dill

**Per Batch**
Calories: 1747; Total Fat: 154g; Carbs: 10g; Net Carbs: 10g; Fiber: 0g; Protein: 83g

**Per Serving**
Calories: 437; Total Fat: 39g; Carbs: 3g; Net Carbs: 3g; Fiber: 0g; Protein: 21g

1. Preheat the oven to 375°F. Coat a 9-by-13-inch baking pan with the butter.

2. In a large bowl, whisk the eggs and cream together. Season with pink Himalayan salt and pepper, and whisk to blend.

3. Pour the egg mixture into the prepared pan. Sprinkle the pancetta in and distribute evenly throughout.

4. Tear off pieces of the prosciutto and place on top, then sprinkle with the dill.

5. Bake for about 25 minutes, or until the edges are golden and the eggs are just set.

6. Transfer to a rack to cool for 5 minutes.

7. Cut into 4 portions and serve hot.

*COOKING TIP* You can use a greased muffin tin with this recipe to create individual egg bites. Just make sure to evenly distribute all the ingredients among the muffin cups.

## VARIATIONS

The great part about a frittata is that you can add so many other ingredients to it. Here are a few variations you can try, but have fun coming up with your own combinations from whatever is in your fridge:

- Browned sausage and fresh spinach.
- Chopped bacon, sliced fresh mushrooms, and fresh spinach.
- Sliced black olives, sliced red peppers, and chopped fresh parsley.
- Diced ham, sliced green peppers, and sliced scallions.

# SAUSAGE BREAKFAST STACKS

The best part about making keto-friendly breakfasts is how many simple ingredients can be combined to give you the perfect healthy fat–filled meal. Sausage patties topped with mashed avocado and a gooey, sunny-side-up egg is the perfect start to a morning.

**30-MINUTE**

**SERVES 2**
**PREP** 10 minutes
**COOK** 15 minutes

8 ounces ground pork

½ teaspoon garlic powder

½ teaspoon onion powder

2 tablespoons ghee, divided

2 large eggs

1 avocado

Pink Himalayan salt

Freshly ground black pepper

**Per Batch**
Calories: 1066; Total Fat: 88g; Carbs: 14g; Net Carbs: 5g; Fiber: 9g; Protein: 57g

**Per Serving**
Calories: 533; Total Fat: 44g; Carbs: 7g; Net Carbs: 3g; Fiber: 5g; Protein: 29g

1. Preheat the oven to 375°F.

2. In a medium bowl, mix well to combine the ground pork, garlic powder, and onion powder. Form the mixture into 2 patties.

3. In a medium skillet over medium-high heat, melt 1 tablespoon of ghee.

4. Add the sausage patties and cook for 2 minutes on each side, until browned.

5. Transfer the sausage to a baking sheet. Cook in the oven for 8 to 10 minutes, until cooked through.

6. Add the remaining 1 tablespoon of ghee to the skillet. When it is hot, crack the eggs into the skillet and cook without disturbing for about 3 minutes, until the whites are opaque and the yolks have set.

7. Meanwhile, in a small bowl, mash the avocado.

8. Season the eggs with pink Himalayan salt and pepper.

9. Remove the cooked sausage patties from the oven.

10. Place a sausage patty on each of two warmed plates. Spread half of the mashed avocado on top of each sausage patty, and top each with a fried egg. Serve hot.

*SUBSTITUTION TIP* You can use precooked frozen sausage patties for an even quicker breakfast. Just make sure they are sugar-free.

# SPICY BREAKFAST SCRAMBLE

A breakfast scramble is one of those meals you can make with a variety of ingredients. This one is inspired by Mexican flavors, but you can just as easily make one with Italian- or Mediterranean-inspired flavors. The Mexican chorizo, a spicy sausage, provides the zesty meat base to this scramble, and with creamy eggs, cheese, and scallions, this easy breakfast will keep you satisfied for hours. I use pepper Jack cheese for extra spice.

**30-MINUTE**

**SERVES 2**
**PREP** 5 minutes
**COOK** 10 minutes

2 tablespoons ghee

6 ounces Mexican chorizo or other spicy sausage

6 large eggs

2 tablespoons heavy (whipping) cream

Pink Himalayan salt

Freshly ground black pepper

½ cup shredded cheese, like pepper Jack, divided

½ cup chopped scallions, white and green parts

**Per Batch**
Calories: 1700; Total Fat: 139g; Carbs: 13g; Net Carbs: 11g; Fiber: 1g; Protein: 91g

**Per Serving**
Calories: 850; Total Fat: 70g; Carbs: 7g; Net Carbs: 6g; Fiber: 1g; Protein: 46g

1. In a large skillet over medium-high heat, melt the ghee. Add the sausage and sauté, browning for about 6 minutes, until cooked through.

2. In a medium bowl, whisk the eggs until frothy.

3. Add the cream, and season with pink Himalayan salt and pepper. Whisk to blend thoroughly.

4. Leaving the fat in the skillet, push the sausage to one side. Add the egg mixture to the other side of the skillet and heat until almost cooked through, about 3 minutes.

5. When the eggs are almost done, mix in half of the shredded cheese.

6. Mix the eggs and sausage together in the skillet. Top with the remaining shredded cheese and the scallions.

7. Spoon onto two plates and serve hot.

*SUBSTITUTION TIP*  If you can't find Mexican chorizo, you can use regular ground beef and spices like garlic powder, cumin, and oregano.

**VARIATIONS**
To take this scramble to the next level, you can add some toppings that will elevate the flavor profile and add healthy fat:

- Top the scramble with ½ sliced avocado, a diced jalapeño, and a dollop of sour cream.
- Top the scramble with 1 tablespoon of salsa, 1 tablespoon of sliced black olives, and 1 tablespoon of chopped fresh cilantro leaves.

# BACON-JALAPEÑO EGG CUPS

Bacon egg cups are the perfect keto breakfast, snack, or even side dish. The crispy bacon on the outside, mixed with the creamy egg middle and spicy jalapeño, will start your day with a kick. The cream cheese mixed with bits of jalapeño pepper provides just the right amount of heat.

**30-MINUTE**

Makes 6 egg cups
**PREP** 5 minutes
**COOK** 25 minutes

**FOR THE BACON**

6 bacon slices

1 tablespoon butter

**FOR THE EGGS**

2 jalapeño peppers

4 large eggs

2 ounces cream cheese, at room temperature

Pink Himalayan salt

Freshly ground black pepper

¼ cup shredded Mexican blend cheese

**Per Batch**
Calories: 955; Total Fat: 80g; Carbs: 7g; Net Carbs: 6g; Fiber: 1g; Protein: 53g

**Per Serving**
Calories: 159; Total Fat: 13g; Carbs: 1g; Net Carbs: 0g; Fiber: 0g; Protein: 9g

**TO MAKE THE BACON**

1. Preheat the oven to 375°F.

2. While the oven is warming up, heat a large skillet over medium-high heat. Add the bacon slices and cook partially, about 4 minutes. Transfer the bacon to a paper towel–lined plate.

3. Coat six cups of a standard muffin tin with the butter. Place a partially cooked bacon strip in each cup to line the sides.

**TO MAKE THE EGGS**

1. Cut one jalapeño lengthwise, seed it, and mince it. Cut the remaining jalapeño into rings, discarding the seeds. Set aside.

2. In a medium bowl, beat the eggs with a hand mixer until well beaten. Add the cream cheese and diced jalapeño, season with pink Himalayan salt and pepper, and beat again to combine.

3. Pour the egg mixture into the prepared muffin tin, filling each cup about two-thirds of the way up so they have room to rise.

4. Top each cup with some of the shredded cheese and a ring of jalapeño, and bake for 20 minutes.

5. Cool for 10 minutes, and serve hot.

*SUBSTITUTION TIP* If you don't have jalapeños available, or you don't like spicy food, you can use bell peppers or another vegetable with a little crunch, like asparagus.

# BACON AND EGG CAULIFLOWER HASH

You don't need potatoes to make a delicious breakfast hash. Cauliflower, a low-carb vegetable, makes a great substitute. In this hash recipe, I've made the classic bacon-and-egg breakfast into an easy, complete, one-skillet breakfast.

**30-MINUTE**
**ONE PAN**

**SERVES 2**
**PREP** 5 minutes
**COOK** 15 minutes

6 bacon slices

½ head cauliflower, cut into small florets

2 garlic cloves, minced

1 medium onion, diced

4 large eggs

1 tablespoon olive oil, if needed

Pink Himalayan salt

Freshly ground black pepper

**Per Batch**
Calories: 790; Total Fat: 54g; Carbs: 29g; Net Carbs: 21g; Fiber: 8g; Protein: 50g

**Per Serving**
Calories: 395; Total Fat: 27g; Carbs: 15g; Nets Carbs: 11g; Fiber: 4g; Protein: 25g

1. In a large skillet over medium-high heat, cook the bacon on both sides until crispy, about 8 minutes. Transfer the bacon to a paper towel–lined plate to drain and cool for 5 minutes. Transfer to a cutting board, and chop the bacon.

2. Turn the heat down to medium, and add the cauliflower, garlic, and onion to the bacon grease in the skillet. Sauté for 5 minutes. If the pan gets dry, add the olive oil. You want the cauliflower florets to just begin to brown before you add the eggs.

3. Using a spoon, make 4 wells in the mixture in the skillet, and crack an egg into each well. Season the eggs and hash with pink Himalayan salt and pepper. Cook the eggs until they set, about 3 minutes.

4. Sprinkle the diced bacon onto the hash mixture, and serve hot.

*INGREDIENT TIP* I buy precut cauliflower florets at Trader Joe's to save time and kitchen prep.

# BACON, SPINACH, AND AVOCADO EGG WRAP

One morning I was planning to make an omelet when the idea of creating an egg wrap came to mind. The egg mixture is cooked like a flat omelet and acts like a crêpe or a tortilla to enclose the other ingredients. You can get creative with the wrapped ingredients; in this case I used bacon, spinach, and avocado.

**30-MINUTE**

**SERVES 2**
**PREP** 10 minutes
**COOK** 10 minutes

6 bacon slices

2 large eggs

2 tablespoons heavy (whipping) cream

Pink Himalayan salt

Freshly ground black pepper

1 tablespoon butter, if needed

1 cup fresh spinach (or other greens of your choice)

½ avocado, sliced

**Per Batch**
Calories: 672; Total Fat: 57g;
Carbs: 9g; Net Carbs: 4g;
Fiber: 5g; Protein: 33g

**Per Serving**
Calories: 336; Total Fat: 29g;
Carbs: 5g; Net Carbs: 2g;
Fiber: 3g; Protein: 17g

1. In a medium skillet over medium-high heat, cook the bacon on both sides until crispy, about 8 minutes. Transfer the bacon to a paper towel–lined plate.

2. In a medium bowl, whisk the eggs and cream, and season with pink Himalayan salt and pepper. Whisk again to combine.

3. Add half the egg mixture to the skillet with the bacon grease.

4. Cook the egg mixture for about 1 minute, or until set, then flip with a spatula and cook the other side for 1 minute.

5. Transfer the cooked-egg mixture to a paper towel–lined plate to soak up extra grease.

6. Repeat steps 4 and 5 for the other half of the egg mixture. If the pan gets dry, add the butter.

7. Place a cooked egg mixture on each of two warmed plates. Top each with half of the spinach, bacon, and avocado slices.

8. Season with pink salt and pepper, and roll the wraps. Serve hot.

*SUBSTITUTION TIP* You can also make these wraps dairy-free, without the heavy cream. Just add an extra egg.

**VARIATIONS**
Egg wraps provide an easy base for many different flavor combinations:

- Chopped romaine lettuce provides a nice crunch to go with the traditional bacon and tomato.
- For extra spice, add diced jalapeños or hot sauce to your egg mixture, along with sausage links and shredded cheese.

# SMOKED SALMON AND CREAM CHEESE ROLL-UPS

Salmon roll-ups are usually considered appetizers, but they also make a delicious breakfast. These are inspired by bagels and lox, but without the carbohydrates.

**30-MINUTE**
**ONE POT**
**NO COOK**

**SERVES 2**
**PREP** 25 minutes

4 ounces cream cheese, at room temperature

1 teaspoon grated lemon zest

1 teaspoon Dijon mustard

2 tablespoons chopped scallions, white and green parts

Pink Himalayan salt

Freshly ground black pepper

1 (4-ounce) package cold-smoked salmon (about 12 slices)

1. Put the cream cheese, lemon zest, mustard, and scallions in a food processor (or blender), and season with pink Himalayan salt and pepper. Process until fully mixed and smooth.

2. Spread the cream-cheese mixture on each slice of smoked salmon, and roll it up. Place the rolls on a plate seam-side down.

3. Serve immediately or refrigerate, covered in plastic wrap or in a lidded container, for up to 3 days.

*SUBSTITUTION TIP* You can substitute chopped fresh dill or capers for the scallions.

**Per Batch**
Calories: 536; Total Fat: 44g;
Carbs: 8g; Net Carbs: 6g;
Fiber: 2g; Protein: 28g

**Per Serving**
Calories: 268; Total Fat: 22g;
Carbs: 4g; Net Carbs: 3g;
Fiber: 1g; Protein: 14g

# BRUSSELS SPROUTS, BACON, AND EGGS

I'm guessing Brussels sprouts haven't been on your breakfast menu before? They didn't use to be on mine either, but now I love them any time of day. When mixed with eggs and bacon, they make a perfect breakfast that is healthy, beautiful, and super easy to make.

**30-MINUTE**

**SERVES 2**
**PREP** 5 minutes
**COOK** 20 minutes

½ pound Brussels sprouts, cleaned, trimmed, and halved

1 tablespoon olive oil

Pink Himalayan salt

Freshly ground black pepper

Nonstick cooking spray

6 bacon slices, diced

4 large eggs

Pinch red pepper flakes

2 tablespoons grated Parmesan cheese

**Per Batch**
Calories: 802; Total Fat: 57g; Carbs: 23g; Net Carbs: 14g; Fiber: 9g; Protein: 54g

**Per Serving**
Calories: 401; Total Fat: 29g; Carbs: 12g; Net Carbs: 7g; Fiber: 5g; Protein: 27g

1. Preheat the oven to 400°F.

2. In a medium bowl, toss the halved Brussels sprouts in the olive oil, and season with pink Himalayan salt and pepper.

3. Coat a 9-by-13-inch baking pan with cooking spray.

4. Put the Brussels sprouts and bacon in the pan, and roast for 12 minutes.

5. Take the pan out of the oven, and stir the Brussels sprouts and bacon. Using a spoon, create 4 wells in the mixture.

6. Carefully crack an egg into each well.

7. Season the eggs with pink Himalayan salt, black pepper, and red pepper flakes.

8. Sprinkle the Parmesan cheese over the Brussels sprouts and eggs.

9. Cook in the oven for 8 more minutes, or until the eggs are cooked to your preference, and serve.

*SUBSTITUTION TIP* You can omit the Parmesan cheese and use your favorite chopped salted nuts instead.

# BLT BREAKFAST SALAD

Salads are not just for lunch or dinner. A hearty salad can be an amazing way to start any day, and salads are quick and easy to put together. Personally, I can eat an oozing, gooey egg on anything, and mixed with the creamy avocado and crunchy bacon, it is the perfect way to start a day.

**30-MINUTE**

**SERVES 2**
**PREP** 10 minutes
**COOK** 5 minutes

2 large eggs

5 ounces organic mixed greens

2 tablespoons olive oil

Pink Himalayan salt

Freshly ground black pepper

1 avocado, thinly sliced

5 grape tomatoes, halved

6 bacon slices, cooked and chopped

**Per Batch**
Calories: 890; Total Fat: 77g; Carbs: 36g; Net Carbs: 7g; Fiber: 12g; Protein: 36g

**Per Serving**
Calories: 445; Total Fat: 39g; Carbs: 18g; Net Carbs: 4g; Fiber: 6g; Protein: 18g

1. In a small saucepan filled with water over high heat, bring the water to a boil. Put the eggs on to softboil, turn the heat down to medium-high, and cook for about 6 minutes.

2. While the eggs are cooking, toss the mixed greens with the olive oil and season with pink Himalayan salt and pepper. Divide the dressed greens between two bowls.

3. Top the greens with the avocado slices, grape tomatoes, and bacon.

4. When the eggs are done, peel them, halve them, and place two halves on top of each salad. Season with more pink Himalayan salt
and pepper and serve.

*SUBSTITUTION TIP* Fresh spinach, or fresh kale trimmed and stemmed and massaged with olive oil to tenderize it, would also be a delicious base for this salad.

# CHEESY EGG AND SPINACH NEST

Cheesy egg nests are one of the easiest but most visually impressive breakfasts you can make. In the skillet, surround a couple of sunny-side-up eggs with cheese to combine a crispy cheese edge with a gooey egg yolk. I've topped the nest with avocado, spinach, and Parmesan cheese for a delicious mixture of flavor and texture.

30-MINUTE
ONE PAN
VEGETARIAN

**SERVES 1**
**PREP** 5 minutes
**COOK** 10 minutes

1 tablespoon olive oil

2 large eggs

Pink Himalayan salt

Freshly ground
black pepper

½ cup shredded
mozzarella cheese

½ avocado, diced

¼ cup chopped
fresh spinach

1 tablespoon grated
Parmesan cheese

**Per Serving**
Calories: 563; Total Fat: 46g;
Carbs: 9g; Net Carbs: 4g;
Fiber: 5g; Protein: 31g

1. In a medium skillet over medium-high heat, heat the olive oil.

2. Crack the eggs into the skillet right next to each other.

3. Season the eggs with pink Himalayan salt and pepper.

4. When the egg whites start to set, after about 2 minutes, sprinkle the mozzarella cheese around the entire perimeter of the eggs.

5. Add the diced avocado and chopped spinach to the cheese "nest."

6. Sprinkle the Parmesan cheese over the eggs and the nest.

7. Cook until the edges of the mozzarella cheese just begin to brown and get crispy, 7 to 10 minutes.

8. Transfer to a warm plate and enjoy hot.

*SUBSTITUTION TIP* You can use fresh flat-leaf Italian parsley instead of spinach.

# KALE-AVOCADO EGG SKILLET

This skillet meal uses mushrooms and kale to provide a hearty base to the healthy fats in eggs and avocado. One-skillet egg dishes are a favorite of mine because I love the way all the flavors come together. Using low-carb vegetables instead of high-starch choices will give you a nourishing start to your day, without heaviness.

30-MINUTE
VEGETARIAN

**SERVES 2**
**PREP** 5 minutes
**COOK** 10 minutes

2 tablespoons olive oil, divided

2 cups sliced mushrooms

5 ounces fresh kale, stemmed and sliced into ribbons

1 avocado, sliced

4 large eggs

Pink Himalayan salt

Freshly ground black pepper

**Per Batch**
Calories: 813; Total Fat: 68g; Carbs: 26g; Net Carbs: 12g; Fiber: 13g; Protein: 35g

**Per Serving**
Calories: 407; Total Fat: 34g; Carbs: 13g; Net Carbs: 6g; Fiber: 7g; Protein: 18g

1. In a large skillet over medium heat, heat 1 tablespoon of olive oil.

2. Add the mushrooms to the pan, and sauté for about 3 minutes.

3. In a medium bowl, massage the kale with the remaining 1 tablespoon of olive oil for 1 to 2 minutes to help tenderize it. Add the kale to the skillet on top of the mushrooms, then place the slices of avocado on top of the kale.

4. Using a spoon, create 4 wells for the eggs. Crack one egg into each well. Season the eggs and kale with pink Himalayan salt and pepper.

5. Cover the skillet and cook for about 5 minutes, or until the eggs reach your desired degree of doneness.

6. Serve hot.

*SUBSTITUTION TIP* You can add asparagus, tomatoes, or another keto-friendly vegetable to the kale if you wish.

# EGG-IN-A-HOLE BREAKFAST BURGER

A burger for breakfast is just plain fun and feels a little rebellious. And everyone knows a gooey egg makes any burger better! Vital Farms Pasture-Raised Eggs are my favorite. This burger is topped with crispy bacon, melted Cheddar cheese, and spicy Sriracha Mayo (page 170) for the perfect breakfast feast. If I haven't made any Sriracha Mayo, I often use Spicy Red Pepper Miso Mayo, which is dairy-free.

**30-MINUTE**
**ONE PAN**

**SERVES 2**
**PREP** 5 minutes
**COOK** 15 minutes

4 bacon slices

6 ounces ground beef

Pink Himalayan salt

Freshly ground
black pepper

2 tablespoons butter

2 large eggs

2 slices Cheddar cheese

1 tablespoon Sriracha Mayo
(page 170)

**Per Batch**
Calories: 1155; Total Fat: 95g;
Carbs: 3g; Net Carbs: 3g;
Fiber: 0g; Protein: 68g

**Per Serving**
Calories: 578; Total Fat: 48g;
Carbs: 2g; Net Carbs: 2g;
Fiber: 0g; Protein: 34g

1. In a large skillet over medium-high heat, cook the bacon on both sides until crispy, about 8 minutes. Transfer the bacon to a paper towel–lined plate.

2. Form the ground beef into two burger patties. Use a small glass or cookie cutter to cut out the middle of each (like a donut). Take the cut-out meat and add it to the edges of the two burgers. Season the meat with pink Himalayan salt and pepper.

3. In the skillet still set over medium-high heat, melt the butter. Add the burger patties, cook the first side for 2 minutes, and then flip.

4. Crack an egg into the middle of each burger, and cook until the whites are set, 1 to 2 minutes. Season the eggs with pink Himalayan salt and pepper.

5. Top each egg with 1 slice of Cheddar cheese, turn the heat off, and cover the skillet to melt the cheese, about 2 minutes.

6. Transfer the burgers to two plates, top each with two bacon slices and some of the sriracha mayo, and serve.

*SUBSTITUTION TIP* You can replace the Cheddar cheese with avocado and the butter with olive oil if you are not eating dairy.

# CREAM CHEESE AND COCONUT FLOUR PANCAKES OR WAFFLES

I experimented with several cream-cheese pancake recipes before I settled on this one. These pancakes have that authentic, puffy pancake feel. You can use the batter on a skillet or griddle for pancakes or in a waffle iron for waffles.

**30-MINUTE**

**VEGETARIAN**

**SERVES 2** (6 pancakes, 3 waffles)
**PREP** 5 minutes
**COOK** 10 minutes

4 large eggs

4 ounces cream cheese, at room temperature

1 teaspoon liquid stevia

1½ teaspoons baking powder

4 tablespoons coconut flour

4 tablespoons butter, divided

Nonstick cooking spray (for waffles)

**Per Batch**
Calories: 1208; Total Fat: 109g; Carbs: 26g; Net Carbs: 16g; Fiber: 10g; Protein: 36g

**Per Serving**
Calories: 604; Total Fat: 55g; Carbs: 13g; Net Carbs: 8g; Fiber: 5g; Protein: 18g

**TO MAKE PANCAKES**

1. In a food processor (or blender), process the eggs, cream cheese, stevia, baking powder, and coconut flour until thoroughly combined.

2. Mix in some add-ins (see Variations) if desired.

3. In a large skillet over medium-high heat, melt 2 tablespoons of butter, turning the skillet to spread it evenly in the bottom of the pan.

4. Pour the batter into the skillet in ¼-cup portions for 3 (4-inch) pancakes.

5. The pancakes will get puffy when it is time to flip them, after about 2 minutes. (They won't really get the air bubbles like a typical pancake, but they will set.) Cook for about 1 minute more, until lightly browned on the bottom.

6. Repeat with the remaining 2 tablespoons of butter for the remaining batter.

7. Serve hot.

**TO MAKE WAFFLES**

1. Preheat the closed waffle iron until it's nice and hot on medium-high heat.

2. In a food processor (or blender), process the eggs, cream cheese, stevia, baking powder, and coconut flour until thoroughly combined.

3. Mix in the add-ins (see Variations) if desired.

4. Open your waffle iron, and spray the top and bottom with nonstick cooking spray.

5. Pour in the batter in three portions, to not quite cover the waffle-iron surface; don't get it close to the edges, or it will spill out when it cooks.

6. Waffles are done when they quit steaming and are lightly browned and crisp. The time will vary depending on your waffle iron.

7. Serve hot.

## VARIATIONS

Use one or more of the following variations to customize your pancakes or waffles with seasonings or add-ins for a truly fabulous treat:

- 2 teaspoons of vanilla extract and a sprinkle of cinnamon. I add these every time I make this pancake-and-waffle mix. I love ground cinnamon, so I add about 1 teaspoon, but you can add as much (or as little) as you want.
- Lily's Dark Chocolate Premium Baking Chips.
- Berries: Blackberries and raspberries are lowest in carbohydrates.
- Crush ½ cup of pork rinds and fold them into the mix. Sounds a little weird, right? But it is delicious, and the pork rinds give the batter a bit more saltiness and a little crunch that's especially nice in waffles.
- Add 1 to 2 tablespoons of your favorite nut butter to the mix to give your pancakes a unique flavor. Brands like Legendary Foods or Buff Bake have some particularly delicious flavors.
- Syrup: I use Walden Farms Calorie-Free Pancake Syrup. They have a blueberry variety that I like, too. I heat up the syrup with 1 tablespoon of butter to add some richness. Sometimes I even mix the maple and blueberry together—yum! But in my opinion, warm syrup is a thousand times better than cold syrup; I heat it in a small saucepan over low heat.

# PANCAKE "CAKE"

Pancakes without any standing over the skillet or griddle while you're flipping? Sign me up! This recipe uses my Cream Cheese and Coconut Flour Pancake recipe (page 35), but in a larger batch cooked in the oven. The result is a light, puffy pancake "cake" that you can top with butter and low-carb syrup. If you want to add additional seasonings or ingredients, see the Variations on page 36.

**30-MINUTE**
**VEGETARIAN**

**SERVES 4**
**PREP** 5 minutes
**COOK** 20 minutes

4 tablespoons butter, plus more for the pan and the top of the cake

8 large eggs

8 ounces cream cheese, at room temperature

4 teaspoons liquid stevia

3 teaspoons baking powder

½ cup coconut flour

**Per Batch**
Calories: 2009; Total Fat: 172g; Carbs: 51g; Net Carbs: 31g; Fiber: 20g; Protein: 72g

**Per Serving**
Calories: 502; Total Fat: 43g; Carbs: 13g; Net Carbs: 8g; Fiber: 5g; Protein: 18g

1. Preheat the oven to 425°F. Coat a 9-by-13-inch baking pan with butter.

2. In a food processor (or blender), process the eggs, cream cheese, stevia, baking powder, and coconut flour until thoroughly combined.

3. Mix in some add-ins (see Variations, page 36), if desired.

4. Spread out the 4 tablespoons of butter in the prepared pan.

5. Put the pan in the oven for 2 to 3 minutes to melt the butter. Let the butter bubble, but make sure it doesn't brown or burn. Remove from the oven.

6. Pour the batter into the pan.

7. Bake for about 15 minutes, or until a paring knife stuck into the center of the cake comes out clean.

8. Place the cake on a cooling rack, and melt a few more tablespoons of butter on top if you wish.

9. Cut the pancake "cake" into 4 pieces and serve warm.

*INGREDIENT TIP* I always add 2 teaspoons of vanilla extract and 2 teaspoons of ground cinnamon to my cake mix, no matter what.

# BREAKFAST QUESADILLA

My daughter absolutely loves breakfast quesadillas. If I let her, she would eat them every single day, but I usually make them once a week. You could use scrambled eggs, but I like to use fried eggs instead so there is some gooey egg yolk in the middle. For this recipe, I use Mission Whole Wheat Low-Carb Tortillas, with 4 net carbs per tortilla.

**30-MINUTE**
**ONE PAN**

**SERVES 2**
**PREP** 5 minutes
**COOK** 20 minutes

2 bacon slices

2 large eggs

Pink Himalayan salt

Freshly ground
black pepper

1 tablespoon olive oil

2 low-carbohydrate tortillas

1 cup shredded Mexican
blend cheese, divided

½ avocado, thinly sliced

**Per Batch**
Calories: 1138; Total Fat: 82g;
Carbs: 53g; Net Carbs: 18g;
Fiber: 35g; Protein: 54g

**Per Serving**
Calories: 569; Total Fat: 41g;
Carbs: 27g; Net Carbs: 9g;
Fiber: 18g; Protein: 27g

1. In a medium skillet over medium-high heat, cook the bacon on both sides until crispy, about 8 minutes. Transfer the bacon to a paper towel–lined plate to drain and cool for 5 minutes. Transfer to a cutting board, and chop the bacon.

2. Turn the heat down to medium, and crack the eggs onto the hot skillet with the bacon grease. Season with pink Himalayan salt and pepper.

3. Cook the eggs for 3 to 4 minutes, until the egg whites are set. If you want the yolks to set, you can cook them longer. Transfer the cooked eggs to a plate.

4. Pour the olive oil into the hot skillet. Place the first tortilla in the pan.

5. Add ½ cup of cheese, place slices of avocado on the cheese in a circle, top with both fried eggs, the chopped bacon, and the remaining ½ cup of cheese, and cover with the second tortilla.

6. Once the cheese starts melting and the bottom of the tortilla is golden, after about 3 minutes, flip the quesadilla. Cook for about 2 minutes on the second side, until the bottom is golden.

7. Cut the quesadilla into slices with a pizza cutter or a chef's knife and serve.

*SUBSTITUTION TIP* If you have Tajín, a seasoning mix, you can use that instead of pink Himalayan salt and pepper for a nice kick of chiles, lime, and salt.

# CREAM CHEESE MUFFINS

I came up with this recipe by serendipity. I intended to make sour-cream muffins, but I was out of sour cream, so I decided to substitute cream cheese mixed with heavy whipping cream. They were so delicious, I've enjoyed this recipe often since then.

30-MINUTE
VEGETARIAN

Makes 6 muffins
**PREP** 10 minutes
**COOK** 10 minutes

4 tablespoons melted butter, plus more for the muffin tin

1 cup almond flour

¾ tablespoon baking powder

2 large eggs, lightly beaten

2 ounces cream cheese mixed with 2 tablespoons heavy (whipping) cream

Handful shredded Mexican blend cheese

**Per Batch**
Calories: 1483; Total Fat: 139g; Carbs: 34g; Net Carbs: 22g; Fiber: 12g; Protein: 45g

**Per Serving**
Calories: 247; Total Fat: 23g; Carbs: 6g; Net Carbs: 4g; Fiber: 2g; Protein: 8g

1. Preheat the oven to 400°F. Coat six cups of a muffin tin with butter.

2. In a small bowl, mix together the almond flour and baking powder.

3. In a medium bowl, mix together the eggs, cream cheese–heavy cream mixture, shredded cheese, and 4 tablespoons of the melted butter.

4. Pour the flour mixture into the egg mixture, and beat with a hand mixer until thoroughly mixed.

5. Pour the batter into the prepared muffin cups.

6. Bake for 12 minutes, or until golden brown on top, and serve.

*SUBSTITUTION TIP* You can use almond meal instead of almond flour. The mix will just have more texture because almond meal is less refined.

**VARIATIONS**
This cream-cheese muffin mix is a great base for savory or sweet additions.

- Add savory Trader Joe's Everything But the Bagel Seasoning on top of the muffins prior to baking to give them a salty, sesame-seed flavor and texture.
- Add diced jalapeños to the mix for a spicy muffin.
- Add 1 tablespoon of grated lemon zest and a handful of blueberries to the mix for a sweeter muffin.

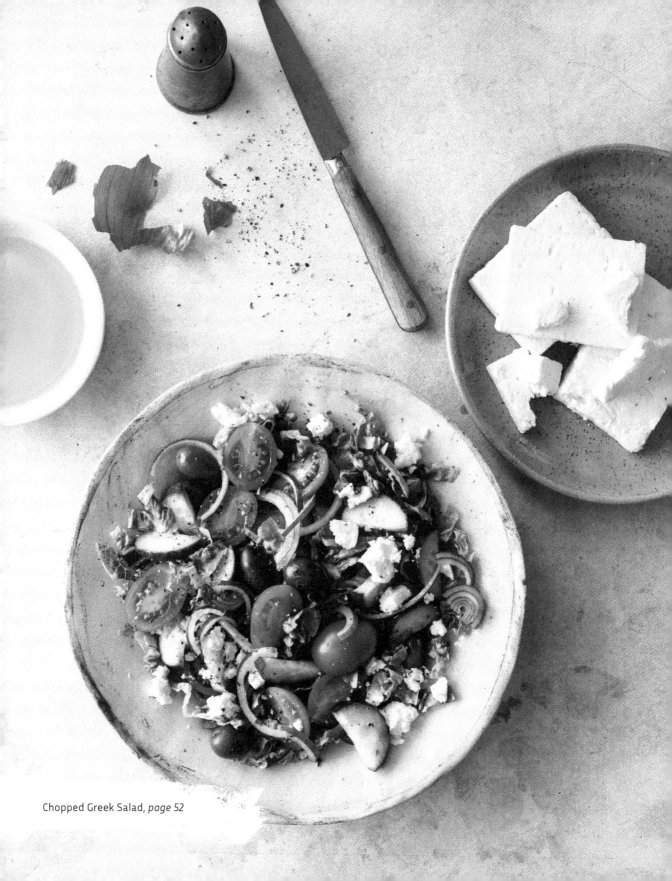

Chopped Greek Salad, *page 52*

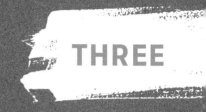

THREE

# HEARTY SOUPS & SALADS

Salads can be your best friend when you are on a ketogenic diet. You just have to know what to watch out for. A lot of restaurant salads or prepackaged convenience salads are loaded with sugar. Sometimes that sugar comes in the form of high-sugar fruit or dried fruit, and sometimes it is in the form of a sweet dressing or candied nuts. Stick to lots of greens, healthy fats, low-carb vegetables, high-fat nuts, and low-carb dressings. These 5 ingredients will really pack your salads full of the optimal amount of taste and nutrition.

Regarding soups, there are a lot of options for the keto dieter: If you are looking for something hearty and filling, choose cream-, cheese-, and cauliflower-based soups. I have been making the Creamy Tomato-Basil Soup in this chapter since "BK" (before keto), and I still love it—simple and delicious.

# CREAMY TOMATO-BASIL SOUP

My parents always request that I make this soup whenever I go to visit them. The soup is so fresh and creamy, you will never want to eat canned soup again.

**30-MINUTE**
**VEGETARIAN**

**SERVES 4**
**PREP** 5 minutes
**COOK** 15 minutes

1 (14.5-ounce) can diced tomatoes (I use Muir Glen Organic Tomatoes with Italian Seasonings)

2 ounces cream cheese

¼ cup heavy (whipping) cream

4 tablespoons butter

¼ cup chopped fresh basil leaves

Pink Himalayan salt

Freshly ground black pepper

**Per Batch**
Calories: 957; Total Fat: 87g; Carbs: 36g; Net Carbs: 29g; Fiber: 6g; Protein: 12g

**Per Serving**
Calories: 239; Total Fat: 22g; Carbs: 9g; Net Carbs: 7g; Fiber: 2g; Protein: 3g

1. Pour the tomatoes with their juices into a food processor (or blender) and purée until smooth.

2. In a medium saucepan over medium heat, cook the tomatoes, cream cheese, heavy cream, and butter for 10 minutes, stirring occasionally, until all is melted and thoroughly combined.

3. Add the basil, and season with pink Himalayan salt and pepper.
Continue stirring for 5 minutes more, until completely smooth. If you wish, you could also use an immersion blender to make short work of smoothing the soup.

4. Pour the soup into four bowls and serve.

*INGREDIENT TIP* You could also use plain, unseasoned diced tomatoes, but I prefer packing in more flavor by using the Italian-seasoned tomatoes.

# BROCCOLI-CHEESE SOUP

When the temperature falls below 60°F in Los Angeles, I always crave a hearty soup. Broccoli-Cheese Soup is one of those keto-perfect soups that make a complete entrée. Tasty and very filling.

30-MINUTE
ONE POT
VEGETARIAN

**SERVES 4**
**PREP** 5 minutes
**COOK** 20 minutes

2 tablespoons butter

1 cup broccoli florets, finely chopped

1 cup heavy (whipping) cream

1 cup chicken or vegetable broth

Pink Himalayan salt

Freshly ground black pepper

1 cup shredded cheese, some reserved for topping (I use sharp Cheddar)

**Per Batch**
Calories: 1533; Total Fat: 149g; Carbs: 17g; Net Carbs: 15g; Fiber: 2g; Protein: 40g

**Per Serving**
Calories: 383; Total Fat: 37g; Carbs: 4g; Net Carbs: 4g; Fiber: 1g; Protein: 10g

1. In a medium saucepan over medium heat, melt the butter.

2. Add the broccoli and sauté in the butter for about 5 minutes, until tender.

3. Add the cream and the chicken broth, stirring constantly. Season with pink Himalayan salt and pepper. Cook, stirring occasionally, for 10 to 15 minutes, until the soup has thickened.

4. Turn down the heat to low, and begin adding the shredded cheese. Reserve a small handful of cheese for topping the bowls of soup. (Do not add all the cheese at once, or it may clump up.) Add small amounts, slowly, while stirring constantly.

5. Pour the soup into four bowls, top each with the reserved cheese, and serve.

*INGREDIENT TIP* If you prefer a smoother texture, you can use an immersion blender for the soup mixture before you add the cheese.

### VARIATIONS
This soup is a creamy, delicious canvas for additional flavors and textures:

- If you like your soup with a spicy kick, you can add ¼ teaspoon of red pepper flakes.
- For additional flavor, add 1 garlic clove, minced, and ¼ onion, diced, when you add the broccoli.
- Crumbled bacon (2 cooked slices) provides a tasty topping for the soup. Sprinkle it over the top.

# CHEESY CAULIFLOWER SOUP

Cauliflower can be used in seemingly anything. Soup is no exception. This is a keto take on a potato soup, minus all of those carbohydrates.

**ONE POT**
**30-MINUTE**

**SERVES 4**
**PREP** 5 minutes
**COOK** 20 minutes

1 tablespoon butter

½ onion, chopped

2 cups riced/shredded cauliflower (I buy it pre-riced at Trader Joe's)

1 cup chicken broth

2 ounces cream cheese

1 cup heavy (whipping) cream

Pink Himalayan salt

Freshly ground pepper

½ cup shredded Cheddar cheese (I use sharp Cheddar)

**Per Batch**
Calories: 1486; Total Fat: 140g; Carbs: 34g; Net Carbs: 24g; Fiber: 10g; Protein: 34g

**Per Serving**
Calories: 372; Total Fat: 35g; Carbs: 9g; Net Carbs: 6g; Fiber: 3g; Protein: 9g

1. In a medium saucepan over medium heat, melt the butter. Add the onion and cook, stirring occasionally, until softened, about 5 minutes.

2. Add the cauliflower and chicken broth, and allow the mixture to come to a boil, stirring occasionally.

3. Lower the heat to medium-low and simmer until the cauliflower is soft enough to mash, about 10 minutes.

4. Add the cream cheese, and mash the mixture.

5. Add the cream and purée the mixture with an immersion blender (or you can pour the soup into the blender, blend it, and then pour it back into the pan and reheat it a bit).

6. Season the soup with pink Himalayan salt and pepper.

7. Pour the soup into four bowls, top each with the shredded Cheddar cheese, and serve.

*INGREDIENT TIP* You could use cauliflower florets instead of riced cauliflower, but you will need to simmer the mixture longer before mashing it, 15 to 20 minutes. You could also use vegetable broth instead of chicken broth for a vegetarian soup.

**VARIATIONS**
As with any creamy soup, crunchy ingredients added on top can be a perfect contrast:

- Add crumbled bacon and chopped scallions atop the soup along with the cheese.
- Add hot sauce for an extra kick.

# TACO SOUP

This soup has a nice kick of flavor from the taco seasoning mixed with the seasoned tomatoes. The base is creamy and rich. It's so rich, you could even make some low-carb tortilla chips and dip them into this delicious mixture. Browning the ground beef on the stove top contributes extra flavor to the soup.

**SERVES 4**
**PREP** 5 minutes
**COOK** 4 hours 10 minutes

1 pound ground beef

Pink Himalayan salt

Freshly ground
black pepper

2 cups beef broth (I use
Kettle & Fire Bone Broth)

1 (10-ounce) can diced
tomatoes (I use Rotel)

1 tablespoon taco
seasoning

8 ounces cream cheese

**Per Batch**
Calories: 1689; Total Fat: 132g;
Carbs: 22g; Net Carbs: 19g;
Fiber: 3g; Protein: 99g

**Per Serving**
Calories: 422; Total Fat: 33g;
Carbs: 6g; Net Carbs: 5g;
Fiber: 1g; Protein: 25g

1. With the crock insert in place, preheat the slow cooker to low.

2. On the stove top, in a medium skillet over medium-high heat, sauté the ground beef until browned, about 8 minutes, and season with pink Himalayan salt and pepper.

3. Add the ground beef, beef broth, tomatoes, taco seasoning, and cream cheese to the slow cooker.

4. Cover and cook on low for 4 hours, stirring occasionally.

5. Ladle into four bowls and serve.

*INGREDIENT TIP* Instead of ground beef, you can use spicy sausage.

# COCONUT AND CAULIFLOWER CURRY SHRIMP SOUP

The Asian flavors in this dish work on all levels: You have the spiciness of the red curry paste along with the creamy fat of coconut milk. Then the juicy shrimp and fresh cilantro finish off the dish.

**ONE POT**

**SERVES 4**

**PREP** 5 minutes

**COOK** 2 hours 15 minutes

8 ounces water

1 (13.5-ounce) can unsweetened full-fat coconut milk

2 cups riced/shredded cauliflower (I buy it pre-riced at Trader Joe's)

2 tablespoons red curry paste

2 tablespoons chopped fresh cilantro leaves, divided

Pink Himalayan salt

Freshly ground black pepper

1 cup shrimp (I use defrosted Trader Joe's Frozen Medium Cooked Shrimp, which are peeled and deveined, with tail off)

**Per Batch**
Calories: 1074; Total Fat: 85g; Carbs: 31g; Net Carbs: 18g; Fiber: 13g; Protein: 64g

**Per Serving**
Calories: 269; Total Fat: 21g; Carbs: 8g; Net Carbs: 5g; Fiber: 3g; Protein: 16g

1. With the crock insert in place, preheat the slow cooker to high.

2. Add the water, coconut milk, riced cauliflower, red curry paste, and 1 tablespoon of chopped cilantro, and season with pink Himalayan salt and pepper. Stir to combine.

3. Cover and cook on high for 2 hours.

4. Season the shrimp with pink Himalayan salt and pepper, add them to the slow cooker, and stir. Cook for an additional 15 minutes.

5. Ladle the soup into four bowls, top each with the remaining chopped cilantro, and serve.

*INGREDIENT TIP* You could also make this soup with cooked, shredded chicken breast.

# ROASTED BRUSSELS SPROUTS SALAD WITH PARMESAN

The difference between this dish and most roasted Brussels sprouts is that here we are just using the leaves of the sprouts, which makes the dish super light. Hazelnuts are not an ingredient I use often, but they really play a starring role in this salad.

30-MINUTE
VEGETARIAN

**SERVES 2**
**PREP** 10 minutes
**COOK** 15 minutes

1 pound Brussels sprouts
1 tablespoon olive oil
Pink Himalayan salt
Freshly ground
black pepper
¼ cup shaved or grated
Parmesan cheese
¼ cup whole, skinless
hazelnuts

**Per Batch**
Calories: 573; Total Fat: 37g;
Carbs: 46g; Net Carbs: 26g;
Fiber: 20g; Protein: 27g

**Per Serving**
Calories: 287; Total Fat: 19g;
Carbs: 23g; Net Carbs: 13g;
Fiber: 10g; Protein: 14g

1. Preheat the oven to 350°F. Line a baking sheet with a silicone baking mat or parchment paper.

2. Trim the bottom and core from each Brussels sprout with a small knife. This will release the leaves. (You can reserve the cores to roast later if you wish.)

3. Put the leaves in a medium bowl; you can use your hands to fully release all the leaves.

4. Toss the leaves with the olive oil and season with pink Himalayan salt and pepper.

5. Spread the leaves in a single layer on the baking sheet. Roast for 10 to 15 minutes, or until lightly browned and crisp.

6. Divide the roasted Brussels sprouts leaves between two bowls, top each with the shaved Parmesan cheese and hazelnuts, and serve.

*SUBSTITUTION TIP* If you don't have hazelnuts, use chopped almonds.

# BLT WEDGE SALAD

To me, a crisp iceberg lettuce wedge topped with chunky blue cheese dressing is delicious on its own. But when you add juicy grape tomatoes and crunchy bacon? It's just perfect.

**30-MINUTE**
**ONE PAN**

**SERVES 2**
**PREP** 10 minutes
**COOK** 10 minutes

4 bacon slices

½ head iceberg lettuce, halved

2 tablespoons blue cheese salad dressing (I use Trader Joe's Chunky Blue Cheese Dressing)

¼ cup blue cheese crumbles

½ cup halved grape tomatoes

**Per Batch**
Calories: 555; Total Fat: 40g;
Carbs: 18g; Net Carbs: 13g;
Fiber: 6g; Protein: 30g

**Per Serving**
Calories: 278; Total Fat: 20g;
Carbs: 9g; Net Carbs: 7g;
Fiber: 3g; Protein: 15g

1. In a large skillet over medium-high heat, cook the bacon on both sides until crispy, about 8 minutes. Transfer the bacon to a paper towel–lined plate to drain and cool for 5 minutes. Transfer to a cutting board, and chop the bacon.

2. Place the lettuce wedges on two plates. Top each with half of the blue cheese dressing, the blue cheese crumbles, the halved grape tomatoes, and the chopped bacon, and serve.

*INGREDIENT TIP* If you have a grill, you can drizzle each of your iceberg lettuce wedges with 1 tablespoon of olive oil, season with pink Himalayan salt and pepper, and grill each side for about 1 minute to add some smoky flavor. Then dress the lettuce wedges as instructed.

# MEXICAN EGG SALAD

I have always been a big fan of egg salad. It also makes a great base for experimentation with different flavors and textures. This version of avocado egg salad brings fresh cilantro and diced jalapeños to the party for a little kick. Then for some crunch, let's put the egg salad on cheese chips! For additional zest, add ½ teaspoon of Tajín seasoning salt and the juice of ½ lime to the egg salad.

**30-MINUTE
VEGETARIAN**

**SERVES 2**
**PREP** 15 minutes
**COOK** 10 minutes

**FOR THE HARDBOILED EGGS**

4 large eggs

**FOR THE CHEESE CHIPS**

½ cup shredded cheese
(I use Mexican blend),
divided

**FOR THE MEXICAN EGG SALAD**

1 jalapeño

1 avocado, halved

Pink Himalayan salt

Freshly ground
black pepper

2 tablespoons chopped
fresh cilantro

**Per Batch**
Calories: 718; Total Fat: 57g;
Carbs: 15g; Net Carbs: 6g;
Fiber: 10g; Protein: 41g

**Per Serving**
Calories: 359; Total Fat: 29g;
Carbs: 8g; Net Carbs: 3g;
Fiber: 5g; Protein: 21g

1. Preheat the oven to 350°F.

2. Line a baking sheet with parchment paper or a silicone baking mat.

**TO MAKE THE HARDBOILED EGGS**

1. In a medium saucepan, cover the eggs with water. Place over high heat, and bring the water to a boil. Once it is boiling, turn off the heat, cover, and leave on the burner for 10 to 12 minutes.

2. Use a slotted spoon to remove the eggs from the pan and run them under cold water for 1 minute or submerge in an ice bath.

3. Gently tap the shells and peel. (I like to run cold water over my hands as I peel the shells off.)

**TO MAKE THE CHEESE CHIPS**

1. While the eggs are cooking, put 2 (¼-cup) mounds of shredded cheese on the prepared pan and bake for about 7 minutes, or until the edges are brown and the middle has fully melted.

2. Remove the cheese chips from the oven and allow to cool for 5 minutes; they will be floppy when they first come out but will crisp as they cool.

**TO MAKE THE MEXICAN EGG SALAD**

1. In a medium bowl, chop the hardboiled eggs.

2. Stem, rib, seed, and dice the jalapeño, and add it to the eggs.

3. Mash the avocado with a fork. Season with pink salt and pepper. Add the avocado and cilantro to the eggs, and stir to combine.

4. Place the cheese chips on two plates, top with the egg salad, and serve.

# BLUE CHEESE AND BACON KALE SALAD

I love a massaged kale salad. Massaging the kale leaves with olive oil breaks down the fibers and makes the greens more tender and easier to digest. Top the kale with bacon, blue cheese crumbles, and pecans, and you have a nutritious salad packed with unique flavors and textures.

30-MINUTE

**SERVES 2**
**PREP** 10 minutes
**COOK** 10 minutes

4 bacon slices

2 cups stemmed and chopped fresh kale

1 tablespoon vinaigrette salad dressing (I use Primal Kitchen Greek Vinaigrette)

Pinch pink Himalayan salt

Pinch freshly ground black pepper

¼ cup pecans

¼ cup blue cheese crumbles

**Per Batch**
Calories: 706; Total Fat: 58g;
Carbs: 20g; Net Carbs: 14g;
Fiber: 5g; Protein: 31g

**Per Serving**
Calories: 353; Total Fat: 29g;
Carbs: 10g; Net Carbs: 7g;
Fiber: 3g; Protein: 16g

1. In a medium skillet over medium-high heat, cook the bacon on both sides until crispy, about 8 minutes. Transfer the bacon to a paper towel–lined plate.

2. Meanwhile, in a large bowl, massage the kale with the vinaigrette for 2 minutes. Add the pink Himalayan salt and pepper. Let
the kale sit while the bacon cooks, and it will get even softer.

3. Chop the bacon and pecans, and add them to the bowl. Sprinkle in the blue cheese.

4. Toss well to combine, portion onto two plates, and serve.

*SUBSTITUTION TIP* Chopped almonds can replace the chopped pecans.

# CHOPPED GREEK SALAD

A Greek salad is one of my restaurant favorites. It is so fresh and easy to make. This one has just a few ingredients, but feel free to get creative with yours.

30-MINUTE
ONE POT
NO COOK
VEGETARIAN

**SERVES 2**
**PREP** 10 minutes

2 cups chopped romaine

½ cup halved grape tomatoes

¼ cup sliced black olives (like Kalamata)

¼ cup feta cheese crumbles

2 tablespoons vinaigrette salad dressing (I use Primal Kitchen Greek Vinaigrette)

Pink Himalayan salt

Freshly ground black pepper

1 tablespoon olive oil

**Per Batch**
Calories: 404; Total Fat: 38g; Carbs: 8g; Net Carbs: 5g; Fiber: 3g; Protein: 7g

**Per Serving**
Calories: 202; Total Fat: 19g; Carbs: 4g; Net Carbs: 3g; Fiber: 2g; Protein: 4g

1. In a large bowl, combine the romaine, tomatoes, olives, feta cheese, and vinaigrette.

2. Season with pink Himalayan salt and pepper, drizzle with the olive oil, and toss to combine.

3. Divide the salad between two bowls and serve.

*SUBSTITUTION TIP* You could replace the feta cheese with goat cheese.

## VARIATIONS

With Greek salad, there are so many great flavors you can add:

- Red onion or finely chopped cucumbers for additional crunch and freshness, and chopped pepperoncini for a zesty kick.
- Finely chopped Genoa salami and pepperoni are good choices.

# MEDITERRANEAN CUCUMBER SALAD

I love making this salad because it is so simple, so delicious, and so packed with fresh flavors. The black olives and feta cheese add some healthy fats, while the cucumbers and tomatoes add that pop of freshness. A great side salad for any Mediterranean-inspired meat dish.

30-MINUTE
ONE POT
VEGETARIAN

**SERVES 2**
**PREP** 10 minutes

1 large cucumber, peeled and finely chopped

½ cup halved grape tomatoes

¼ cup halved black olives (I use Kalamata)

¼ cup crumbled feta cheese

Pink Himalayan salt

Freshly ground black pepper

2 tablespoons vinaigrette salad dressing (I use Primal Kitchen Greek Vinaigrette)

**Per Batch**
Calories: 303; Total Fat: 25g;
Carbs: 11g; Net Carbs: 8g;
Fiber: 3g; Protein: 8g

**Per Serving**
Calories: 152; Total Fat: 13g;
Carbs: 6g; Net Carbs: 4g;
Fiber: 2g; Protein: 4g

1. In a large bowl, combine the cucumber, tomatoes, olives, and feta cheese. Season with pink Himalayan salt and pepper. Add the dressing and toss to combine.

2. Divide the salad between two bowls and serve.

*INGREDIENT TIP* This salad can be eaten immediately, of course, but I think it is even better if you cover it with wrap and put it in the fridge to let the dressing marinate the salad ingredients for a few hours.

# AVOCADO EGG SALAD LETTUCE CUPS

I just recently started making egg salad with avocado instead of mayo. It adds a delicious flavor element. And for some enjoyable crunch, add sliced radishes.

30-MINUTE
VEGETARIAN

**SERVES 2**
**PREP** 15 minutes
**COOK** 15 minutes

**FOR THE HARDBOILED EGGS**

4 large eggs

**FOR THE EGG SALAD**

1 avocado, halved

Pink Himalayan salt

Freshly ground
black pepper

½ teaspoon freshly
squeezed lemon juice

4 butter lettuce cups,
washed and patted dry with
paper towels or a clean
dish towel

2 radishes, thinly sliced

**Per Batch**
Calories: 515; Total Fat: 40g;
Carbs: 15g; Net Carbs: 5g;
Fiber: 10g; Protein: 29g

**Per Serving**
Calories: 258; Total Fat: 20g;
Carbs: 8g; Net Carbs: 3g;
Fiber: 5g; Protein: 15g

**TO MAKE THE HARDBOILED EGGS**

1. In a medium saucepan, cover the eggs with water. Place over high heat, and bring the water to a boil. Once it is boiling, turn off the heat, cover, and leave on the burner for 10 to 12 minutes.

2. Remove the eggs with a slotted spoon and run them under cold water for 1 minute or submerge them in an ice bath.

3. Then gently tap the shells and peel. Run cold water over your hands as you remove the shells.

**TO MAKE THE EGG SALAD**

1. In a medium bowl, chop the hardboiled eggs.

2. Add the avocado to the bowl, and mash the flesh with a fork. Season with pink Himalayan salt and pepper, add the lemon juice, and stir to combine.

3. Place the 4 lettuce cups on two plates. Top the lettuce cups with the egg salad and the slices of radish and serve.

*SUBSTITUTION TIP* You could also use romaine hearts or baby cos lettuce.

**VARIATIONS**

For this recipe, you can incorporate additional ingredients that you may have in your refrigerator or pantry:

- Add a guacamole vibe to your egg salad with chopped jalapeño and red onion.
- Chopped bacon adds appealing texture to your egg salad, or add slices of crisp bacon to your lettuce cups.

# AVOCADO CAPRESE SALAD

Caprese salads are a classic. For a keto twist, I add avocado for additional healthy fats, and arugula for a peppery flavor. These ingredients make the dish super filling, too.

30-MINUTE
NO COOK
VEGETARIAN

**SERVES 2**
**PREP** 5 minutes

2 cups arugula

1 tablespoon olive oil, divided

Pink Himalayan salt

Freshly ground black pepper

1 avocado, sliced

4 fresh mozzarella balls, sliced

1 Roma tomato, sliced

4 fresh basil leaves, cut into ribbons

**Per Batch**
Calories: 640; Total Fat: 54g; Carbs: 20g; Net Carbs: 9g; Fiber: 11g; Protein: 25g

**Per Serving**
Calories: 320; Total Fat: 27g; Carbs: 10g; Net Carbs: 5g; Fiber: 6g; Protein: 13g

1. In a large bowl, toss the arugula with ½ tablespoon of olive oil and season with pink Himalayan salt and pepper.

2. Divide the arugula between two plates.

3. Top the arugula with the avocado, mozzarella, and tomatoes, and drizzle with the remaining ½ tablespoon of olive oil. Season with pink Himalayan salt and pepper.

4. Sprinkle the basil on top and serve.

*SUBSTITUTION TIP* For an extra kick of flavor, you can replace the olive oil with a vinaigrette dressing. I use Primal Kitchen Greek Vinaigrette.

# SHRIMP AND AVOCADO SALAD

This salad needs to chill for a bit before serving, but waiting that extra time is well worth it. To make the recipe super easy, I buy cooked and peeled shrimp, but you can choose whichever kind of shrimp you like.

**SERVES 2**
**PREP** 5 minutes, plus
30 minutes to chill
**COOK** 2 minutes

1 tablespoon olive oil

1 pound shrimp (I use defrosted Trader Joe's Frozen Medium Cooked Shrimp, which are peeled and deveined, with tail off)

Pink Himalayan salt

Freshly ground black pepper

1 avocado, cubed

1 celery stalk, chopped

¼ cup mayonnaise

1 teaspoon freshly squeezed lime juice

**Per Batch**
Calories: 1141; Total Fat: 81g;
Carbs: 15g; Net Carbs: 5g;
Fiber: 10g; Protein: 100g

**Per Serving**
Calories: 571; Total Fat: 41g;
Carbs: 8g; Net Carbs: 3g;
Fiber: 5g; Protein: 50g

1. In a large skillet over medium heat, heat the olive oil. When the oil is hot, add the shrimp. Cook until they turn pink, 1 to 2 minutes. Season with pink Himalayan salt and pepper.

2. Transfer the shrimp to a medium bowl, cover, and refrigerate.

3. In a medium bowl, combine the avocado, celery, and mayonnaise. Add the lime juice, and season with pink Himalayan salt.
Stir to combine. Add the chilled shrimp, and toss to combine.

4. Cover the salad, and refrigerate to chill for 30 minutes before serving.

*SUBSTITUTION TIP*  For an additional kick, use Tajín seasoning salt instead of regular pink Himalayan salt. Tajín is a Mexican seasoning salt that combines chiles, lime, and sea salt.

**VARIATIONS**
I love the creaminess of this chilled salad. If you have fresh herbs or greens in the refrigerator, you might want to add them:
- Add chopped fresh dill to the salad mixture.
- Scoop the salad mixture onto butter lettuce cups or romaine leaves for added freshness and crunch.

# SALMON CAESAR SALAD

This salad is creamy and full of healthy fats, and it has the salty crunch of bacon. Personally, I love salmon anytime and in any way, so this salad is perfect. Who wouldn't prefer getting crunch from bacon instead of the standard carb-full croutons?

**30-MINUTE**
**ONE PAN**

**SERVES 2**
**PREP** 5 minutes
**COOK** 20 minutes

4 bacon slices

2 (6-ounce) salmon fillets

Pink Himalayan salt

Freshly ground
black pepper

1 tablespoon ghee,
if needed

½ avocado, sliced

2 romaine hearts or 2 cups
chopped romaine

2 tablespoons Caesar
dressing (I use Primal
Kitchen Caesar with
Avocado Oil)

**Per Batch**
Calories: 932; Total Fat: 63g;
Carbs: 11g; Net Carbs: 5g;
Fiber: 7g; Protein: 79g

**Per Serving**
Calories: 466; Total Fat: 32g;
Carbs: 6g; Net Carbs: 3g;
Fiber: 4g; Protein: 40g

1. In a medium skillet over medium-high heat, cook the bacon on both sides until crispy, about 8 minutes. Transfer the bacon to a paper towel–lined plate.

2. Meanwhile, pat the salmon with a paper towel to remove excess water. Season both sides with pink Himalayan salt and pepper.

3. With the bacon grease still in the skillet, add the salmon. If you need more grease in the pan, add the ghee to the bacon grease.

4. Cook the salmon for 5 minutes on each side, or until it reaches your preferred degree of doneness. I like it medium-rare.

5. Tear the bacon into pieces. Season the avocado with pink Himalayan salt and pepper.

6. Divide the romaine, bacon, and avocado between two plates.

7. Top the salads with the salmon fillets, drizzle Caesar dressing on top, and serve.

*INGREDIENT TIP*  You could bake the bacon and salmon instead of using the skillet. Preheat the oven to 400°F, and line a baking sheet with aluminum foil. Place the bacon slices and salmon fillets on the baking sheet together. Bake for 15 minutes, and then broil for 5 minutes, or until the top of the salmon browns.

# SALMON AND SPINACH COBB SALAD

The Cobb salad is a perfect keto food. It's fresh, full of healthy fats, and just plain delicious. I prefer topping mine with salmon rather than the standard turkey or chicken. And I use the warm, gooey egg yolk as a super-flavorful dressing for the salad.

**30-MINUTE**

**SERVES 2**
**PREP** 5 minutes
**COOK** 25 minutes

4 bacon slices

2 large eggs

2 (6-ounce) salmon fillets

Pink Himalayan salt

Freshly ground
black pepper

1 tablespoon ghee,
if needed

1 avocado, sliced

6 ounces organic
baby spinach

¼ cup crumbled
blue cheese

1 tablespoon olive oil

**Per Batch**
Calories: 1251; Total Fat: 85g;
Carbs: 23g; Net Carbs: 10g;
Fiber: 13g; Protein: 107g

**Per Serving**
Calories: 623; Total Fat: 43g;
Carbs: 12g; Net Carbs: 5g;
Fiber: 7g; Protein: 54g

1. In a medium skillet over medium-high heat, cook the bacon on both sides until crispy, about 8 minutes. Transfer the bacon to a paper towel–lined plate.

2. Bring a small saucepan filled with water to a boil over high heat. Put the eggs on to softboil, turn the heat down to medium-high, and cook for about 6 minutes.

3. Meanwhile, pat the salmon fillets on both sides with a paper towel to remove excess moisture. Season both sides with pink Himalayan salt and pepper.

4. With the bacon grease still in the skillet, add the salmon. If you need more grease in the pan, add some ghee to the bacon grease.

5. Cook the salmon on medium-high heat for 5 minutes on each side, or until it reaches your preferred degree of doneness. (I like it medium-rare.)

6.  Meanwhile, transfer the bacon to a cutting board and chop it. Peel the softboiled eggs. Season the avocado with pink Himalayan salt and pepper.

7.  Divide the spinach, bacon, and avocado between two plates.

8.  Carefully halve the softboiled eggs and place them on the salads. Sprinkle the blue cheese crumbles over the salads.

9.  Top with the salmon, drizzle the salads with the olive oil, and serve.

*INGREDIENT TIP*  You could use arugula instead of spinach, or a crunchier green like romaine if you prefer.

**VARIATIONS**

- Add halved grape tomatoes for a pop of acidity and freshness.
- Add sliced black olives for an additional salty element.

# TACO SALAD

Taco salads are perfect for the keto diet if you don't use the taco shell. Making them at home is easy. Just brown some ground beef and combine it with a variety of fresh ingredients.

**30-MINUTE**
**ONE PAN**

**SERVES 2**
**PREP** 10 minutes
**COOK** 10 minutes

1 tablespoon ghee

1 pound ground beef

Pink Himalayan salt

Freshly ground
black pepper

2 cups chopped romaine

1 avocado, cubed

½ cup halved grape
tomatoes

½ cup shredded cheese
(I use Mexican blend)

**Per Batch**
Calories: 1390; Total Fat: 104g;
Carbs: 19g; Net Carbs: 7g;
Fiber: 12g; Protein: 96g

**Per Serving**
Calories: 659; Total Fat: 52g;
Carbs: 10g; Net Carbs: 4g;
Fiber: 6g; Protein: 48g

1. In a large skillet over medium-high heat, heat the ghee.

2. When the ghee is hot, add the ground beef, breaking it up into smaller pieces with a spoon. Stir, cooking until the beef is browned, about 10 minutes. Season with pink Himalayan salt and pepper.

3. Divide the romaine into two bowls. Season with pink Himalayan salt and pepper.

4. Add the avocado and tomatoes, top with the beef and shredded cheese, and serve.

*SUBSTITUTION TIP* You could replace pink Himalayan salt and pepper with taco seasoning.

## VARIATIONS

- Feel free to add a dollop of sour cream and some chopped scallions or jalapeños for crunch and healthy fat.
- You can make your own tortilla strips by cutting a low-carb tortilla into strips, tossing the strips in olive oil, seasoning them with salt and pepper, and baking them in a single layer on a baking sheet for 10 minutes at 425°F.

# CHEESEBURGER SALAD

I love to order a lettuce-wrapped burger when I go to a restaurant, but for some reason I never make them at home. This cheeseburger salad will give you the same taste, all mixed in one bowl. I especially love the pickles in this recipe, so if you want to add more, do it!

**30-MINUTE**

**SERVES 2**
**PREP** 10 minutes
**COOK** 10 minutes

1 tablespoon ghee

1 pound ground beef

Pink Himalayan salt

Freshly ground
black pepper

½ cup finely chopped
dill pickles

2 cups chopped romaine

½ cup shredded
Cheddar cheese

2 tablespoons ranch salad
dressing (I use Primal
Kitchen Ranch)

**Per Batch**
Calories: 1324; Total Fat: 100g;
Carbs: 12g; Net Carbs: 8g;
Fiber: 3g; Protein: 94g

**Per Serving**
Calories: 662; Total Fat: 50g;
Carbs: 6g; Net Carbs: 4g;
Fiber: 2g; Protein: 47g

1. In a medium skillet over medium-high heat, heat the ghee.

2. When the ghee is hot, add the ground beef, breaking it up into smaller pieces with a spoon. Stir, cooking until the beef is browned, about 10 minutes. Season with pink Himalayan salt and pepper.

3. Put the pickles in a large bowl, and add the romaine and cheese.

4. Using a slotted spoon, transfer the browned beef from the skillet to the bowl.

5. Top the salad with the dressing, and toss to thoroughly coat.

6. Divide into two bowls and serve.

*SUBSTITUTION TIP* You could replace the ground beef with ground turkey.

## VARIATIONS

Your favorite burger toppings would also be tasty as toppings on this salad:

- For an extra tone of flavor, add a handful of diced onion to the salad, and 1 teaspoon of yellow mustard and ¼ teaspoon of paprika to the ranch dressing.
- Of course, you can also add chopped bacon.

# CALIFORNIA STEAK SALAD

Avocados and strawberries just scream California. In this recipe, they serve as the perfect companion to the skirt steak and the peppery flavor of arugula.

**30-MINUTE**

**SERVES 2**
**PREP** 15 minutes
**COOK** 10 minutes

8 ounces skirt steak

Pink Himalayan salt

Freshly ground
black pepper

2 tablespoons butter

2 cups arugula

1 tablespoon olive oil

1 avocado, sliced

2 fresh strawberries, sliced

¼ cup slivered,
chopped almonds

**Per Batch**
Calories: 1001; Total Fat: 81g;
Carbs: 21g; Net Carbs: 8g;
Fiber: 13g; Protein: 55g

**Per Serving**
Calories: 501; Total Fat: 41g;
Carbs: 11g; Net Carbs: 4g;
Fiber: 7g; Protein: 28g

1. Heat a large skillet over high heat.

2. Pat the steak dry with a paper towel, and season both sides with pink Himalayan salt and pepper.

3. Add the butter to the skillet. When it melts, put the steak in the skillet.

4. Sear the steak for about 3 minutes on each side, for medium-rare.

5. Transfer the steak to a cutting board and let rest for at least 5 minutes.

6. In a large bowl, toss the arugula with the olive oil and a pinch each of pink Himalayan salt and pepper.

7. Divide the arugula between two plates, and top with the sliced avocado, strawberries, and almonds.

8. Slice the skirt steak across the grain, top the salads with it, and serve.

*SUBSTITUTION TIP* Flank steak would work just as well as skirt steak. You can also use sliced cold leftover steak, which works beautifully.

# SKIRT STEAK COBB SALAD

Skirt steak is the perfect choice for topping a salad because it cooks quickly and is flavorful. Cook the skirt steak just to medium-rare to keep it tender, and cut it against the grain when serving. This salad doesn't call for marinating the steak ahead of time, but you can if you prefer. I find that rubbing the steak with pink Himalayan salt and black pepper and cooking it on a screaming hot pan with some oil is perfect.

**30-MINUTE**
**ONE PAN**

**SERVES 2**
**PREP** 15 minutes
**COOK** 10 minutes

8 ounces skirt steak

Pink Himalayan salt

Freshly ground
black pepper

1 tablespoon butter

2 romaine hearts or 2 cups chopped romaine

½ cup halved grape tomatoes

¼ cup crumbled
blue cheese

¼ cup pecans

1 tablespoon olive oil

**Per Batch**
Calories: 902; Total Fat: 71g;
Carbs: 14g; Net Carbs: 9g;
Fiber: 6g; Protein: 60g

**Per Serving**
Calories: 451; Total Fat: 36g;
Carbs: 7g; Net Carbs: 5g;
Fiber: 3g; Protein: 30g

1. Heat a large skillet over high heat.

2. Pat the steak dry with a paper towel, and season both sides with pink Himalayan salt and pepper.

3. Add the butter to the skillet. When it melts, put the steak in the skillet.

4. Sear the steak for about 3 minutes on each side, for medium-rare.

5. Transfer the steak to a cutting board and let it rest for at least 5 minutes.

6. Meanwhile, divide the romaine between two plates, and top with the grape tomato halves, blue cheese, and pecans. Drizzle with the olive oil.

7. Slice the skirt steak across the grain, top the salads with it, and serve.

*SUBSTITUTION TIP* Flank steak works just as well as skirt steak.

**VARIATIONS**
Salads are the perfect canvas for creativity when it comes to toppings. I generally look in my refrigerator and see what I have on hand. These options are just some of the great additions available:
- Balsamic dressing and a sliced hardboiled egg.
- Walnuts in place of the pecans, and 1 sliced avocado.

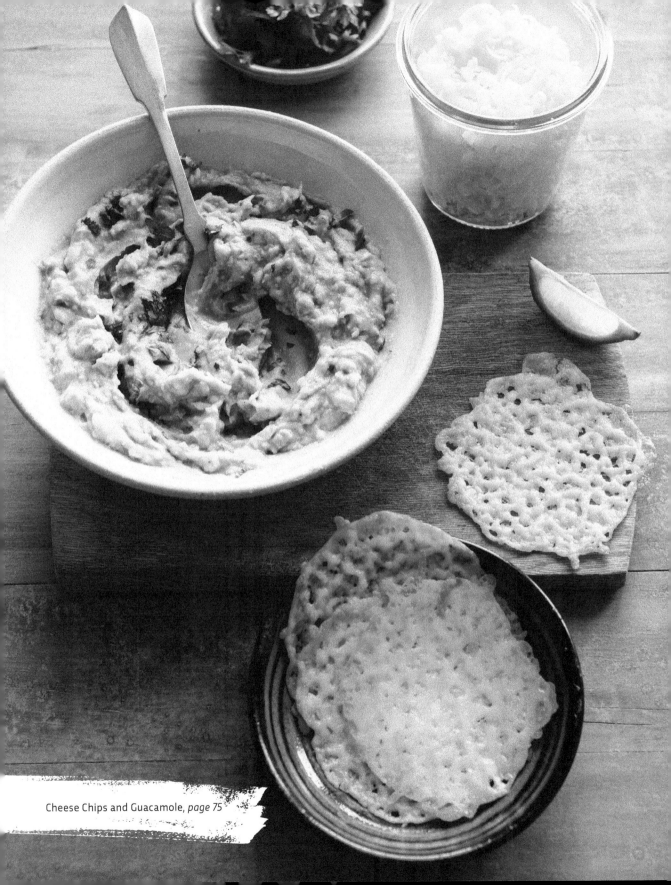

Cheese Chips and Guacamole, *page 75*

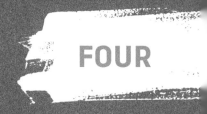

# FOUR

# SIDE DISHES & SNACKS

These side dishes are some of my absolute favorite keto recipes. I love them because they are super easy to make and they combine some fun flavors. I often eat one of these as my main dish when I am craving a veggie-forward meal, but they are also great beside your favorite protein. This chapter really highlights some of the many creative ways you can use vegetables on a keto diet.

# ROASTED CAULIFLOWER WITH PROSCIUTTO, CAPERS, AND ALMONDS

This dish is one of my favorite things to eat. Sometimes I eat it as my dinner, but it is also perfect as a side with any meat. The capers are probably the best part; they provide a nice pop of flavor, and the slivered almonds give it a surprising crunch. I always make roasted cauliflower right after I make bacon, because I have all that wonderful bacon grease left in the pan, and the cauliflower soaks it right up. Sometimes I also throw a couple of seasoned chicken breasts into the pan with the cauliflower for a complete meal in one pan.

30-MINUTE
ONE PAN

**SERVES 2**
**PREP** 5 minutes
**COOK** 25 minutes

12 ounces cauliflower florets (I get precut florets at Trader Joe's)

2 tablespoons leftover bacon grease, or olive oil

Pink Himalayan salt

Freshly ground black pepper

2 ounces sliced prosciutto, torn into small pieces

¼ cup slivered almonds

2 tablespoons capers

2 tablespoons grated Parmesan cheese

**Per Batch**
Calories: 576; Total Fat: 48g; Carbs: 14g; Net Carbs: 7g; Fiber: 6g; Protein: 28g

**Per Serving**
Calories: 288; Total Fat: 24g; Carbs: 7g; Net Carbs: 4g; Fiber: 3g; Protein: 14g

1. Preheat the oven to 400°F. Line a baking pan with a silicone baking mat or parchment paper.

2. Put the cauliflower florets in the prepared baking pan with the bacon grease, and season with pink Himalayan salt and pepper. Or if you are using olive oil instead, drizzle the cauliflower with olive oil and season with pink Himalayan salt and pepper.

3. Roast the cauliflower for 15 minutes.

4. Stir the cauliflower so all sides are coated with the bacon grease.

5. Distribute the prosciutto pieces in the pan. Then add the slivered almonds and capers. Stir to combine. Sprinkle the Parmesan cheese on top, and roast for 10 minutes more.

6. Divide between two plates, using a slotted spoon so you don't get excess grease in the plates, and serve.

*SUBSTITUTION TIP* Sliced green olives work well if you don't have capers.

# BUTTERY SLOW-COOKER MUSHROOMS

There is something about dry ranch-dressing mix that makes such a great seasoning. When I first started cooking, I used it all the time to make chicken, pork chops, and this mushroom dish. Your house will smell incredible while these are cooking in the slow cooker. I love to pop these while I am watching football, but they are also a delicious side dish for most meats. You can easily double or triple this recipe for a larger group.

ONE POT
VEGETARIAN

**SERVES 2**
**PREP** 10 minutes
**COOK** 4 hours

6 tablespoons butter

1 tablespoon packaged dry ranch-dressing mix

8 ounces fresh cremini mushrooms

2 tablespoons grated Parmesan cheese

1 tablespoon chopped fresh flat-leaf Italian parsley

**Per Batch**
Calories: 701; Total Fat: 72g;
Carbs: 9g; Net Carbs: 7g;
Fiber: 2g; Protein: 11g

**Per Serving**
Calories: 351; Total Fat: 36g;
Carbs: 5g; Net Carbs: 4g;
Fiber: 1g; Protein: 6g

1. With the crock insert in place, preheat the slow cooker to low.

2. Put the butter and the dry ranch dressing in the bottom of the slow cooker, and allow the butter to melt. Stir to blend the dressing mix and butter.

3. Add the mushrooms to the slow cooker, and stir to coat with the butter-dressing mixture. Sprinkle the top with the Parmesan cheese.

4. Cover and cook on low for 4 hours.

5. Use a slotted spoon to transfer the mushrooms to a serving dish. Top with the chopped parsley and serve.

*SUBSTITUTION TIP* If you don't have dry ranch-dressing mix, for a similar result you can combine equal amounts of onion powder, garlic powder, dried thyme, pink Himalayan salt, pepper, dried parsley, and a dash of paprika.

# BAKED ZUCCHINI GRATIN

I love a gratin, and potatoes are out of the question, but this cheesy dish with a crispy pork-rind topping will serve as a delicious low-carb alternative. The crushed pork rinds act like a bread-crumb topping, and you can use any flavor of pork rinds you prefer. Simply toss them in the food processor (or blender) for a few seconds to crush. The mixture of the Brie and Gruyère cheeses is what makes this dish so unique!

**SERVES 2**
**PREP** 10 minutes, plus 30 minutes to drain
**COOK** 25 minutes

1 large zucchini, cut into ¼-inch-thick slices

Pink Himalayan salt

1 ounce Brie cheese, rind trimmed off

1 tablespoon butter

Freshly ground black pepper

⅓ cup shredded Gruyère cheese

¼ cup crushed pork rinds

**Per Batch**
Calories: 709; Total Fat: 50g; Carbs: 10g; Net Carbs: 7g; Fiber: 3g; Protein: 55g

**Per Serving**
Calories: 355; Total Fat: 25g; Carbs: 5g; Net Carbs: 4g; Fiber: 2g; Protein: 28g

1. Salt the zucchini slices and put them in a colander in the sink for 45 minutes; the zucchini will shed much of their water.

2. Preheat the oven to 400°F.

3. When the zucchini have been "weeping" for about 30 minutes, in a small saucepan over medium-low heat, heat the Brie and butter, stirring occasionally, until the cheese has melted and the mixture is fully combined, about 2 minutes.

4. Arrange the zucchini in an 8-inch baking dish so the zucchini slices are overlapping a bit. Season with pepper.

5. Pour the Brie mixture over the zucchini, and top with the shredded Gruyère cheese.

6. Sprinkle the crushed pork rinds over the top.

7. Bake for about 25 minutes, until the dish is bubbling and the top is nicely browned, and serve.

*SUBSTITUTION TIP* You can use a crème de Brie soft cheese as well. Some have garlic or other herbs in them, which are tasty additions to this dish.

# ROASTED RADISHES WITH BROWN BUTTER SAUCE

These warm, buttery roasted radishes look and taste like you are eating a baby red potato. They are crispy on the outside, warm and smooth on the inside. The brown butter sauce makes this dish truly delicious.

30-MINUTE
VEGETARIAN

**SERVES 2**
**PREP** 10 minutes
**COOK** 15 minutes

2 cups halved radishes

1 tablespoon olive oil

Pink Himalayan salt

Freshly ground
black pepper

2 tablespoons butter

1 tablespoon chopped fresh
flat-leaf Italian parsley

**Per Batch**
Calories: 361; Total Fat: 37g;
Carbs: 8g; Net Carbs: 4g;
Fiber: 4g; Protein: 2g

**Per Serving**
Calories: 181; Total Fat: 19g;
Carbs: 4g; Net Carbs: 2g;
Fiber: 2g; Protein: 1g

1. Preheat the oven to 450°F.

2. In a medium bowl, toss the radishes in the olive oil and season with pink Himalayan salt and pepper.

3. Spread the radishes on a baking sheet in a single layer. Roast for 15 minutes, stirring halfway through.

4. Meanwhile, when the radishes have been roasting for about 10 minutes, in a small, light-colored saucepan over medium heat, melt the butter completely, stirring frequently, and season with pink Himalayan salt. When the butter begins to bubble and foam, continue stirring. When the bubbling diminishes a bit, the butter should be a nice nutty brown. The browning process should take about 3 minutes total. Transfer the browned butter to a heat-safe container (I use a mug).

5. Remove the radishes from the oven, and divide them between two plates. Spoon the brown butter over the radishes, top with the chopped parsley, and serve.

*INGREDIENT TIP* You can keep the stems on the radishes to roast them if you prefer them that way.

# PARMESAN AND PORK RIND GREEN BEANS

I love green beans. Growing up, we never roasted them, but now that is my favorite way to cook most vegetables. Drizzled in olive oil and seasoned with a bit of salt plus the Parmesan cheese and pork rinds, the roasted beans are bursting with flavor.

30-MINUTE

**SERVES 2**
**PREP** 5 minutes
**COOK** 15 minutes

½ pound fresh green beans

2 tablespoons crushed pork rinds

2 tablespoons olive oil

1 tablespoon grated Parmesan cheese

Pink Himalayan salt

Freshly ground black pepper

**Per Batch**
Calories: 350; Total Fat: 30g;
Carbs: 16g; Net Carbs: 10g;
Fiber: 6g; Protein: 8g

**Per Serving**
Calories: 175; Total Fat: 15g;
Carbs: 8g; Net Carbs: 5g;
Fiber: 3g; Protein: 6g

1. Preheat the oven to 400°F.

2. In a medium bowl, combine the green beans, pork rinds, olive oil, and Parmesan cheese. Season with pink Himalayan salt and
pepper, and toss until the beans are thoroughly coated.

3. Spread the bean mixture on a baking sheet in a single layer, and roast for about 15 minutes. At the halfway point, give the pan a little shake to move the beans around, or just give them a stir.

4. Divide the beans between two plates and serve.

*INGREDIENT TIP* You can use any flavor of pork rinds to add additional zest to the green beans, but I typically use the original flavor.

# PESTO CAULIFLOWER STEAKS

I love making pesto. Anytime I buy a bunch of fresh basil for a recipe, I use the leftovers to make pesto. And I usually opt for whatever nuts I have around. The flavorful pesto paired with the melted cheese is a perfect topping for cauliflower steaks.

**30-MINUTE**
**VEGETARIAN**

**SERVES 2**
**PREP** 5 minutes
**COOK** 20 minutes

2 tablespoons olive oil, plus more for brushing

½ head cauliflower

Pink Himalayan salt

Freshly ground black pepper

2 cups fresh basil leaves

½ cup grated Parmesan cheese

¼ cup almonds

½ cup shredded mozzarella cheese

**Per Batch**
Calories: 895; Total Fat: 68g;
Carbs: 34g; Net Carbs: 20g;
Fiber: 14g; Protein: 47g

**Per Serving**
Calories: 448; Total Fat: 34g;
Carbs: 17g; Net Carbs: 10g;
Fiber: 7g; Protein: 24g

1. Preheat the oven to 425°F. Brush a baking sheet with olive oil or line with a silicone baking mat.

2. To prep the cauliflower steaks, remove and discard the leaves and cut the cauliflower into 1-inch-thick slices. You can roast the extra floret crumbles that fall off with the steaks.

3. Place the cauliflower steaks on the prepared baking sheet, and brush them with the olive oil. You want the surface just lightly coated so it gets caramelized. Season with pink Himalayan salt and pepper.

4. Roast the cauliflower steaks for 20 minutes.

5. Meanwhile, put the basil, Parmesan cheese, almonds, and 2 tablespoons of olive oil in a food processor (or blender), and season with pink Himalayan salt and pepper. Mix until combined.

6. Spread some pesto on top of each cauliflower steak, and top with the mozzarella cheese. Return to the oven and bake until the cheese melts, about 2 minutes.

7. Place the cauliflower steaks on two plates, and serve hot.

*SUBSTITUTION TIP* I use almonds for my pesto instead of the conventional pine nuts because I always seem to have almonds in the house. But if you have pine nuts on hand, you can definitely use those.

# TOMATO, AVOCADO, AND CUCUMBER SALAD

You can assemble this flavorful salad in minutes. It's a perfect dish for a potluck because everyone will enjoy it. I like to use small Persian cucumbers for this salad because they are crisper and have very tiny seeds.

30-MINUTE
NO COOK
VEGETARIAN

**SERVES 2**
**PREP** 5 minutes

½ cup grape
tomatoes, halved

4 small Persian cucumbers
or 1 English cucumber,
peeled and finely chopped

1 avocado, finely chopped

¼ cup crumbled feta cheese

2 tablespoons vinaigrette
salad dressing (I use Primal
Kitchen Greek Vinaigrette)

Pink Himalayan salt

Freshly ground
black pepper

**Per Batch**
Calories: 516; Total Fat: 45g;
Carbs: 23g; Net Carbs: 11g;
Fiber: 12g; Protein: 10g

**Per Serving**
Calories: 258; Total Fat: 23g;
Carbs: 12g; Net Carbs: 6g;
Fiber: 6g; Protein: 5g

1. In a large bowl, combine the tomatoes, cucumbers, avocado, and feta cheese.

2. Add the vinaigrette, and season with pink Himalayan salt and pepper. Toss to thoroughly combine.

3. Divide the salad between two plates and serve.

*SUBSTITUTION TIP* You could replace the feta cheese with goat cheese.

## VARIATIONS
The flavors and textures in this salad pair perfectly with the following additions:
- ½ red onion, finely chopped, for additional crunch and freshness
- Sliced black olives

# CRUNCHY PORK RIND ZUCCHINI STICKS

My daughter isn't a fan of zucchini. But she loves these crunchy, salty zucchini sticks. They make for a delicious side dish for just about any meal.

30-MINUTE

**SERVES 2**
**PREP** 5 minutes
**COOK** 25 minutes

2 medium zucchini, halved lengthwise and seeded

¼ cup crushed pork rinds

¼ cup grated Parmesan cheese

2 garlic cloves, minced

2 tablespoons melted butter

Pink Himalayan salt

Freshly ground black pepper

Olive oil, for drizzling

**Per Batch**
Calories: 461; Total Fat: 39g; Carbs: 15g; Net Carbs: 11g; Fiber: 4g; Protein: 17g

**Per Serving**
Calories: 231; Total Fat: 20g; Carbs: 8g; Net Carbs: 6g; Fiber: 2g; Protein: 9g

1. Preheat the oven to 400°F. Line a baking sheet with aluminum foil or a silicone baking mat.

2. Place the zucchini halves cut-side up on the prepared baking sheet.

3. In a medium bowl, combine the pork rinds, Parmesan cheese, garlic, and melted butter, and season with pink Himalayan salt and pepper. Mix until well combined.

4. Spoon the pork-rind mixture onto each zucchini stick, and drizzle each with a little olive oil.

5. Bake for about 20 minutes, or until the topping is golden brown.

6. Turn on the broiler to finish browning the zucchini sticks, 3 to 5 minutes, and serve.

*INGREDIENT TIP* You can use a spoon to hollow out the zucchini boats if you want to make a bit more room for toppings.

# CHEESE CHIPS AND GUACAMOLE

Chips and guacamole is one of those appetizers you miss when you are on a keto diet. But these cheese chips are so easy to make, there is no reason to miss chips. And you may even like these better!

30-MINUTE
VEGETARIAN

**SERVES 2**
**PREP** 10 minutes
**COOK** 10 minutes

**FOR THE CHEESE CHIPS**

1 cup shredded cheese
(I use Mexican blend)

**FOR THE GUACAMOLE**

1 avocado, mashed

Juice of ½ lime

1 teaspoon diced jalapeño

2 tablespoons chopped
fresh cilantro leaves

Pink Himalayan salt

Freshly ground
black pepper

**Per Batch**
Calories: 646; Total Fat: 54g;
Carbs: 16g; Net Carbs: 6g;
Fiber: 10g; Protein: 30g

**Per Serving**
Calories: 323; Total Fat: 27g;
Carbs: 8g; Net Carbs: 3g;
Fiber: 5g; Protein: 15g

**TO MAKE THE CHEESE CHIPS**

1. Preheat the oven to 350°F. Line a baking sheet with parchment paper or a silicone baking mat.

2. Add ¼-cup mounds of shredded cheese to the pan, leaving plenty of space between them, and bake until the edges are brown and the middles have fully melted, about 7 minutes.

3. Set the pan on a cooling rack, and let the cheese chips cool for 5 minutes. The chips will be floppy when they first come out of the oven but will crisp as they cool.

**TO MAKE THE GUACAMOLE**

1. In a medium bowl, mix together the avocado, lime juice, jalapeño, and cilantro, and season with pink Himalayan salt and pepper.

2. Top the cheese chips with the guacamole, and serve.

*INGREDIENT TIP* You can also add some of the diced jalapeños to the cheese mixture before baking the chips.

# CAULIFLOWER "POTATO" SALAD

This recipe is another great example of how versatile cauliflower is. No one is going to be fooled into thinking this is an actual potato salad, but it is delicious in its own right. Feel free to add in some of the variations to really take it over the top!

**VEGETARIAN**

**SERVES 2**
**PREP** 10 minutes,
plus 3 hours to chill
**COOK** 25 minutes

½ head cauliflower
1 tablespoon olive oil
Pink Himalayan salt
Freshly ground
black pepper
⅓ cup mayonnaise
1 tablespoon mustard
¼ cup diced dill pickles
1 teaspoon paprika

**Per Batch**
Calories: 772; Total Fat: 74g;
Carbs: 26g; Net Carbs: 16g;
Fiber: 10g; Protein: 10g

**Per Serving**
Calories: 386; Total Fat: 37g;
Carbs: 13g; Net Carbs: 8g;
Fiber: 5g; Protein: 5g

1. Preheat the oven to 400°F. Line a baking sheet with aluminum foil or a silicone baking mat.

2. Cut the cauliflower into 1-inch pieces.

3. Put the cauliflower in a large bowl, add the olive oil, season with the pink Himalayan salt and pepper, and toss to combine.

4. Spread the cauliflower out on the prepared baking sheet and bake for 25 minutes, or just until the cauliflower begins to brown. Halfway through the cooking time, give the pan a couple of shakes or stir so all sides of the cauliflower cook.

5. In a large bowl, mix the cauliflower together with the mayonnaise, mustard, and pickles. Sprinkle the paprika on top, and chill in the refrigerator for 3 hours before serving.

*INGREDIENT TIP* You don't want to use precut cauliflower florets because the pieces can be too small or too large and the salad won't have the same "potato salad" feel. Make sure you use bite-size pieces of cauliflower.

**VARIATIONS**
These additions make this delicious salad even tastier:
- Chopped hardboiled eggs on top
- Diced celery and minced white onion added to the mix

# LOADED CAULIFLOWER MASHED "POTATOES"

Cauliflower is definitely a staple in a keto diet. It is very low in carbohydrates and is so versatile. In fact for me, it is just as good as a potato.

**30-MINUTE**

**SERVES 4**
**PREP** 10 minutes
**COOK** 10 minutes

1 head fresh cauliflower, cut into cubes

2 garlic cloves, minced

6 tablespoons butter

2 tablespoons sour cream

Pink Himalayan salt

Freshly ground black pepper

1 cup shredded cheese (I use Colby Jack)

6 bacon slices, cooked and crumbled

**Per Batch**
Calories: 1513; Total Fat: 132g; Carbs: 34g; Net Carbs: 22g; Fiber: 12g; Protein: 58g

**Per Serving**
Calories: 757; Total Fat: 38g; Carbs: 17g; Net Carbs: 11g; Fiber: 6g; Protein: 29g

1. Boil a large pot of water over high heat. Add the cauliflower. Reduce the heat to medium-low and simmer for 8 to 10 minutes, until fork-tender. (You can also steam the cauliflower if you have a steamer basket.)

2. Drain the cauliflower in a colander, and turn it out onto a paper towel–lined plate to soak up the water. Blot to remove any remaining water from the cauliflower pieces. This step is important; you want to get out as much water as possible so the mash won't be runny.

3. Add the cauliflower to the food processor (or blender) with the garlic, butter, and sour cream, and season with pink Himalayan salt and pepper.

4. Mix for about 1 minute, stopping to scrape down the sides of the bowl every 30 seconds.

5. Divide the cauliflower mix evenly among four small serving dishes, and top each with the cheese and bacon crumbles. (The cheese should melt from the hot cauliflower. But if you want to reheat it, you can put the cauliflower in oven-safe serving dishes and pop them under the broiler for 1 minute to heat up the cauliflower and melt the cheese.)

6. Serve warm.

**VARIATIONS**

Anything you would use to top mashed potatoes will work well on mashed cauliflower. Try the following additions:

- Instead of Colby cheese, you can sprinkle ¼ cup of grated Parmesan cheese over the top, with 2 slices of prosciutto, chopped, and 3 tablespoons of chopped chives. For crispy prosciutto, place it under the broiler briefly.

# KETO BREAD

I tried a lot of keto-friendly bread variations until I finally came up with this combination. I love the texture, and it works as a great basic recipe for creating sweet or savory variations.

**30-MINUTE**
**VEGETARIAN**

**MAKES 1 LOAF, 12 SLICES**
**PREP** 5 minutes
**COOK** 25 minutes

5 tablespoons butter, at room temperature, divided

6 large eggs, lightly beaten

1½ cups almond flour

3 teaspoons baking powder

1 scoop MCT oil powder (optional, but it is flavorless and adds high-quality fats; I use Perfect Keto's MCT oil powder)

Pinch pink Himalayan salt

**Per Loaf**
Calories: 1973; Total Fat: 178g; Carbs: 46g; Net Carbs: 27g; Fiber: 19g; Protein: 74g

**Per Slice**
Calories: 165; Total Fat: 15g; Carbs: 4g; Net Carbs: 2g; Fiber: 2g; Protein: 6g

1. Preheat the oven to 390°F. Coat a 9-by-5-inch loaf pan with 1 tablespoon of butter.

2. In a large bowl, use a hand mixer to mix the eggs, almond flour, remaining 4 tablespoons of butter, baking powder, MCT oil powder (if using), and pink Himalayan salt until thoroughly blended. Pour into the prepared pan.

3. Bake for 25 minutes, or until a toothpick inserted in the center comes out clean.

4. Slice and serve.

## VARIATIONS

You may miss bread on the keto diet. In addition to the main recipe, try these variations:

- Keto Pumpkin Bread: Mix all the ingredients together along with ¼ can of pure pumpkin purée. (Make sure you aren't buying sugar-filled pumpkin pie mix; you just want plain pumpkin purée. In my experience, Trader Joe's carries it only seasonally, but you can find it at Target, Safeway, or Walmart year-round.) Also mix in 2 to 3 teaspoons of liquid stevia, depending on how sweet you want it, and 1 tablespoon of pumpkin pie spice (a mixture of cinnamon, nutmeg, ginger, and allspice). Bake according to the recipe instructions.
- Keto Chocolate Chip Bread: Mix the ingredients as instructed, then fold in ½ cup of keto-friendly chocolate chips. I use Lily's, which are sweetened with stevia.

# DEVILED EGGS

I have always been addicted to deviled eggs. I particularly love this recipe, which has sour cream in the egg mixture. This one's a game changer.

**MAKES 24 DEVILED EGGS**
**PREP** 30 minutes
**COOK** 15 minutes

12 large eggs

½ cup mayonnaise

¼ cup sour cream

1 tablespoon
ground mustard

Pink Himalayan salt

Freshly ground
black pepper

1 teaspoon paprika

**Per Batch**
Calories: 1775; Total Fat: 159g;
Carbs: 12g; Net Carbs: 11g;
Fiber: 1g; Protein: 79g

**Per Egg Half**
Calories: 74; Total Fat: 7g;
Carbs: 1g; Net Carbs: 0g;
Fiber: 0g; Protein: 3g

1. To hardboil the eggs, place the eggs in a large saucepan and cover with 3 to 4 inches of water. Bring the water to a boil, turn off the heat, cover the pot, and let sit for 15 minutes. Drain the eggs and fill the pan with ice-cold water (you can add ice cubes, too). One by one, lightly tap the eggs on the countertop to crack and then peel them under cold running water. Put them on a paper towel–lined plate.

2. Halve the eggs lengthwise. With a small spoon, carefully remove the yolks, transfer the yolks to a small bowl, and mash them.

3. Add the mayonnaise, sour cream, and mustard, and season with pink Himalayan salt and pepper. Mix with a fork until smooth.

4. Spoon the yolk mixture back into the indentations in the egg whites, or pipe it in with a cake-decorating bag if you want it to look pretty. Sprinkle with the paprika and serve.

## DEVILED EGGS *continued*

*SIMPLIFYING TIP* My daughter frequently watches YouTube videos, usually DIY or baking videos, and she picks up some awesome tricks! One that I have now adopted is a super-easy way to put mix into a makeshift piping bag. You'll just need a zip-top sandwich bag and a drinking cup. Put the bag in the cup, folding the edges of the bag over the sides of the cup. Spoon the mix into the zip-top bag, lift the bag out of the cup, cut off a small corner, and BOOM! You've created a simple piping bag.

### VARIATIONS

A simple, classic deviled egg is great, but I can't resist taking everything to another level, so I love to add toppings:

- BLT Deviled Eggs: These are my favorite. I have been making them for years—since way before I was keto. Top the egg mixture with crumbled bacon, chopped tomato, and chopped basil, which acts as the "L." Everyone loves them, keto or not!

- Bacon-Jalapeño Deviled Eggs: This version uses the egg mixture with added crumbled bacon and diced jalapeños. Remove the seeds to decrease the heat level.

- Bacon-Avocado Deviled Eggs: Add ½ avocado to the egg mixture along with 1 tablespoon of freshly squeezed lime juice. Then crumble 2 slices of crisply cooked bacon on top. I also like to replace the paprika with Tajín, which is a delicious Mexican seasoning salt made with chiles and lime.

# CHICKEN-PECAN SALAD CUCUMBER BITES

I used to love the Sonoma Chicken Salad at Whole Foods, because the chicken, celery, grapes, and pecans are such a tasty combination. In this recipe I have left out the grapes to make it keto-friendly, and I have added cucumber slices to provide a fresh crunch. This dish is a super-easy light dinner or a perfect appetizer.

30-MINUTE

NO COOK

**SERVES 2**
**PREP** 15 minutes

1 cup diced cooked chicken breast

2 tablespoons mayonnaise

¼ cup chopped pecans

¼ cup diced celery

Pink Himalayan salt

Freshly ground black pepper

1 cucumber, peeled and cut into ¼-inch slices

**Per Batch**
Calories: 646; Total Fat: 47g; Carbs: 12g; Net Carbs: 7g; Fiber: 5g; Protein: 46g

**Per Serving**
Calories: 323; Total Fat: 24g; Carbs: 6g; Net Carbs: 4g; Fiber: 3g; Protein: 23g

1. In a medium bowl, mix together the chicken, mayonnaise, pecans, and celery. Season with pink Himalayan salt and pepper.

2. Lay the cucumber slices out on a plate, and add a pinch of pink Himalayan salt to each.

3. Top each cucumber slice with a spoonful of the chicken-salad mixture and serve.

*INGREDIENT TIP* I have kept these bites wrapped in the refrigerator for 2 days before serving, and they were still fresh and crunchy.

# BUFFALO CHICKEN DIP

This dip is a great side dish for game day. It has all the taste of chicken wings, but in a dip.

**SERVES 2**
**PREP** 10 minutes
**COOK** 20 minutes

Butter or olive oil, for greasing the pan

1 large cooked boneless chicken breast, shredded

8 ounces cream cheese

½ cup shredded Cheddar cheese

½ cup chunky blue cheese dressing

¼ cup buffalo wing sauce (I use Frank's RedHot Sauce)

**Per Batch**
Calories: 1717; Total Fat: 145g;
Carbs: 15g; Net Carbs: 15g;
Fiber: 0g; Protein: 81g

**Per Serving**
Calories: 859; Total Fat: 73g;
Carbs: 8g; Net Carbs: 8g;
Fiber: 0g; Protein: 41g

1. Preheat the oven to 375°F. Grease a small baking pan.

2. In a medium bowl, mix together the chicken, cream cheese, Cheddar cheese, blue cheese dressing, and wing sauce. Transfer the mixture to the prepared baking pan.

3. Bake for 20 minutes.

4. Pour into a dip dish and serve hot.

*SERVING TIP* Pair this dip with celery stalks or pork rinds.

# ROASTED BRUSSELS SPROUTS WITH BACON

I didn't try Brussels sprouts until I was 30 years old! The first time I had them they were roasted, and I realized that I loved Brussels sprouts. This dish is beyond easy because the bacon bits cook while the Brussels sprouts roast, all in just one pan, for a dish that's full of flavor.

30-MINUTE

**SERVES 2**
**PREP** 5 minutes
**COOK** 25 minutes

½ pound Brussels sprouts, cleaned, trimmed, and halved

1 tablespoon olive oil

Pink Himalayan salt

Freshly ground black pepper

1 teaspoon red pepper flakes

6 bacon slices

1 tablespoon grated Parmesan cheese

**Per Batch**
Calories: 496; Total Fat: 36g; Carbs: 21g; Net Carbs: 13g; Fiber: 9g; Protein: 27g

**Per Serving**
Calories: 248; Total Fat: 18g; Carbs: 11g; Net Carbs: 7g; Fiber: 5g; Protein: 14g

1. Preheat the oven to 400°F.

2. In a medium bowl, toss the Brussels sprouts with the olive oil, season with pink Himalayan salt and pepper, and add the red pepper flakes.

3. Cut the bacon strips into 1-inch pieces. (I use kitchen shears.)

4. Place the Brussels sprouts and bacon on a baking sheet in a single layer. Roast for about 25 minutes. About halfway through the baking time, give the pan a little shake to move the sprouts around, or give them a stir. You want your Brussels sprouts crispy and browned on the outside.

5. Remove the Brussels sprouts from the oven. Divide them between two plates, top each serving with Parmesan cheese, and serve.

*INGREDIENT TIP* Just leave out the Parmesan cheese to make this dish dairy-free.

# SALAMI, PEPPERONCINI, AND CREAM CHEESE PINWHEELS

These pinwheels are a great appetizer to bring to a gathering or just to keep in your fridge so that you have keto-friendly bites on hand. Fill the insides of these shapes with just about anything—I have really been enjoying sliced pepperoncini lately, they make any dish so much zestier! Another great thing about this dish is there is no cooking required—you just need some muscle to roll out the cream cheese.

**NO COOK**

**SERVES 2**

**PREP** 20 minutes, plus 6 hours to chill

8 ounces cream cheese, at room temperature

¼ pound salami, thinly sliced

2 tablespoons sliced pepperoncini (I use Mezzetta)

**Per Batch**
Calories: 1166; Total Fat: 107g; Carbs: 13g; Net Carbs: 13g; Fiber: 0g; Protein: 38g

**Per Serving**
Calories: 583; Total Fat: 54g; Carbs: 7g; Net Carbs: 7g; Fiber: 0g; Protein: 19g

1. Lay out a sheet of plastic wrap on a large cutting board or counter.

2. Place the cream cheese in the center of the plastic wrap, and then add another layer of plastic wrap on top. Using a rolling pin, roll the cream cheese until it is even and about ¼ inch thick. Try to make the shape somewhat resemble a rectangle.

3. Pull off the top layer of plastic wrap.

4. Place the salami slices so they overlap to completely cover the cream-cheese layer.

5. Place a new piece of plastic wrap on top of the salami layer so that you can flip over your cream cheese–salami rectangle. Flip the layer so the cream cheese side is up.

6. Remove the plastic wrap and add the sliced pepperoncini in a layer on top.

7. Roll the layered ingredients into a tight log, pressing the meat and cream cheese together. (You want it as tight as possible.) Then wrap the roll with plastic wrap and refrigerate for at least 6 hours so it will set.

8. Use a sharp knife to cut the log into slices and serve.

*INGREDIENT TIP* You could replace the pepperoncini with a variety of things, including chopped dill pickles, scallions, or jalapeños, or sliced bell pepper.

# CAULIFLOWER STEAKS WITH BACON AND BLUE CHEESE

This recipe uses the familiar flavors of a wedge salad. But instead of lettuce, it has a warm, caramelized cauliflower steak as the base. Then it is topped with chunky blue cheese dressing and crispy bacon.

30-MINUTE
ONE PAN
VEGETARIAN

**SERVES 2**
**PREP** 5 minutes
**COOK** 20 minutes

½ head cauliflower

1 tablespoon olive oil

Pink Himalayan salt

Freshly ground
black pepper

4 bacon slices

2 tablespoons blue cheese
salad dressing (I use Trader
Joe's Chunky Blue Cheese
Dressing)

**Per Batch**
Calories: 507; Total Fat: 38g;
Carbs: 22g; Net Carbs: 14g;
Fiber: 8g; Protein: 22g

**Per Serving**
Calories: 254; Total Fat: 19g;
Carbs: 11g; Net Carbs: 7g;
Fiber: 4g; Protein: 11g

1. Preheat the oven to 425°F. Line a baking sheet with aluminum foil or a silicone baking mat.

2. To prep the cauliflower steaks, remove and discard the leaves and cut the cauliflower into 1-inch-thick slices. You can also roast the extra floret crumbles that fall off with the steaks.

3. Place the cauliflower steaks on the prepared baking sheet, and brush with the olive oil. You want the surface just lightly coated with the oil so it gets caramelized. Season with pink Himalayan salt and pepper. Place the bacon slices on the pan, along with the cauliflower floret crumbles.

4. Roast the cauliflower steaks for 20 minutes.

5. Place the cauliflower steaks on two plates. Drizzle with blue cheese dressing, top with crumbled bacon, and serve.

*SUBSTITUTION TIP* You could follow the same instructions to make this dish with cabbage steaks instead of cauliflower.

# BACON-WRAPPED JALAPEÑOS

In the fall and winter, when I am glued to the TV watching my Denver Broncos play, this is my favorite game food! It's so easy to make, with only three ingredients, but they do take a good amount of prep time. (I put my daughter to work prepping the ingredients so I don't miss the game.)

**30-MINUTE**
**ONE PAN**

**SERVES 4**
**PREP** 10 minutes
**COOK** 20 minutes

10 jalapeños

8 ounces cream cheese, at room temperature

1 pound bacon (you will use about half a slice per popper)

**Per Batch**
Calories: 3272; Total Fat: 268g; Carbs: 24g; Net Carbs: 20g; Fiber: 4g; Protein: 183g

**Per Serving**
Calories: 164; Total Fat: 13g; Carbs: 1g; Net Carbs: 1g; Fiber: 0g; Protein: 9g

1. Preheat the oven to 450°F. Line a baking sheet with aluminum foil or a silicone baking mat.

2. Halve the jalapeños lengthwise, and remove the seeds and membranes (if you like the extra heat, leave them in). Place them on the prepared pan cut-side up.

3. Spread some of the cream cheese inside each jalapeño half.

4. Wrap a jalapeño half with a slice of bacon (depending on the size of the jalapeño, use a whole slice of bacon, or half).

5. Secure the bacon around each jalapeño with 1 to 2 tooth-picks so it stays put while baking.

6. Bake for 20 minutes, until the bacon is done and crispy.

7. Serve hot or at room temperature. Either way, they are delicious!

*INGREDIENT TIP* I recommend wearing thin rubber gloves when you are prepping a batch of fresh jalapeños. The chile pepper capsaicin soaks into your skin, and even after washing your hands multiple times, it can still be irritating. It is so easy to forget and touch your eyes or face.

# CREAMY BROCCOLI-BACON SALAD

This fresh, creamy cold salad is the perfect companion for grilled meats, fish, or any summer-friendly entrée. The crunchy raw broccoli is the star, but the honey mustard adds a nice sweet kick to the otherwise salty ingredients.

**SERVES 2**
**PREP** 10 minutes,
plus at least 1 hour to chill
**COOK** 10 minutes

6 bacon slices

½ pound fresh broccoli, cut into small florets

¼ cup sliced almonds

⅓ cup mayonnaise

1 tablespoon honey mustard dressing

**Per Batch**
Calories: 1097; Total Fat: 97g; Carbs: 32g; Net Carbs: 22g; Fiber: 10g; Protein: 32g

**Per Serving**
Calories: 549; Total Fat: 49g; Carbs: 16g; Net Carbs: 11g; Fiber: 5g; Protein: 16g

1. In a large skillet over medium-high heat, cook the bacon on both sides until crispy, about 8 minutes. Transfer the bacon to a paper towel–lined plate to drain and cool for 5 minutes. When cool, break the bacon into crumbles.

2. In a large bowl, combine the broccoli with the almonds and bacon.

3. In a small bowl, mix together the mayonnaise and honey mustard.

4. Add the dressing to the broccoli salad, and toss to thoroughly combine.

5. Chill the salad for 1 hour or more before serving.

*SUBSTITUTION TIP* You can replace the sliced almonds with sunflower seeds.

## VARIATIONS

Consider adding these elements to the salad for a bit of crispness and sweetness:

- ½ red onion, chopped, or 2 scallions, chopped
- 2 carrots, shredded

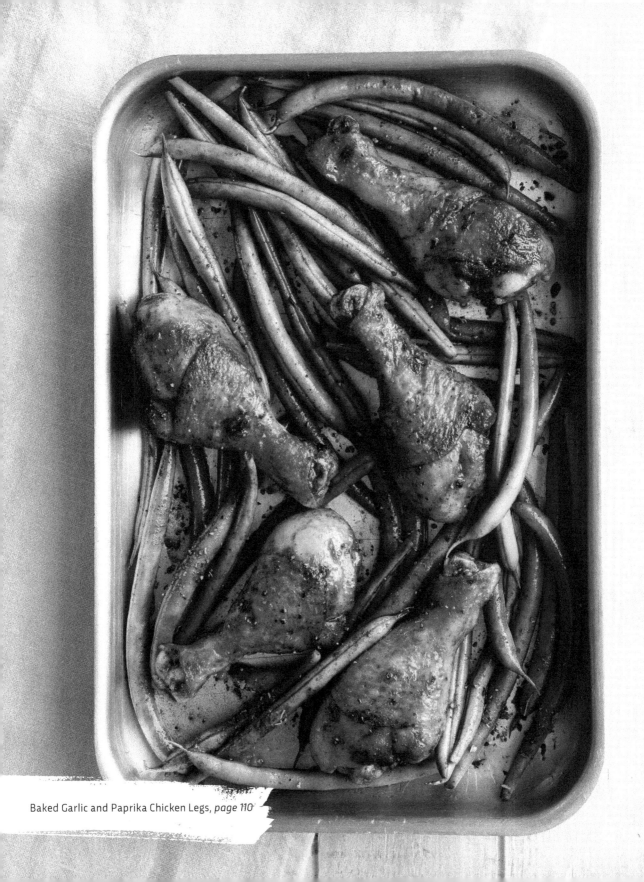

Baked Garlic and Paprika Chicken Legs, *page 110*

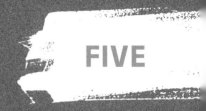

FIVE

# FISH & POULTRY ENTRÉES

Chicken and fish are staples in my house. There are so many ways to add flavor and fat to these proteins to make them extra delicious and perfect for the keto diet. You can enjoy any of these entrées on their own or pair them with a side dish from chapter 4. Whether you are looking for a dish that is crunchy or creamy, this chapter is filled with recipes you'll love to cook over and over again.

# BAKED LEMON-BUTTER FISH

Buttery, flaky fish is something I could eat any day of the week. The lemon provides the bright counterpoint to the mild fish, and the capers give the dish a zesty pop.

30-MINUTE

**SERVES 2**
**PREP** 10 minutes
**COOK** 20 minutes

4 tablespoons butter, plus more for coating

2 (5-ounce) tilapia fillets

Pink Himalayan salt

Freshly ground black pepper

2 garlic cloves, minced

1 lemon, zested and juiced

2 tablespoons capers, rinsed and chopped

**Per Batch**
Calories: 597; Total Fat: 52g; Carbs: 9g; Net Carbs: 6g; Fiber: 2g; Protein: 29g

**Per Serving**
Calories: 299; Total Fat: 26g; Carbs: 5g; Net Carbs: 3g; Fiber: 1g; Protein: 16g

1. Preheat the oven to 400°F. Coat an 8-inch baking dish with butter.

2. Pat dry the tilapia with paper towels, and season on both sides with pink Himalayan salt and pepper. Place in the prepared baking dish.

3. In a medium skillet over medium heat, melt the butter. Add the garlic and cook for 3 to 5 minutes, until slightly browned but not burned.

4. Remove the garlic butter from the heat, and mix in the lemon zest and 2 tablespoons of lemon juice.

5. Pour the lemon-butter sauce over the fish, and sprinkle the capers around the baking pan.

6. Bake for 12 to 15 minutes, until the fish is just cooked through, and serve.

*SUBSTITUTION TIP*  You could use any mild white fish with this recipe. Even salmon is delicious with the lemon-butter sauce.

# FISH TACO BOWL

This Fish Taco Bowl makes the most of just a few ingredients, with exciting punches of chile, lime, and red pepper from the Tajín seasoning salt. The coleslaw mix is a time-saver, and I absolutely love the crunch of the cabbage mixed with the smooth avocado.

**30-MINUTE**

**SERVES 2**
**PREP** 10 minutes
**COOK** 15 minutes

2 (5-ounce) tilapia fillets

1 tablespoon olive oil

4 teaspoons Tajín seasoning salt, divided

2 cups presliced coleslaw cabbage mix

1 tablespoon Spicy Red Pepper Miso Mayo, plus more for serving

1 avocado, mashed

Pink Himalayan salt

Freshly ground black pepper

**Per Batch**
Calories: 629; Total Fat: 47g; Carbs: 23g; Net Carbs: 10g; Fiber: 14g; Protein: 32g

**Per Serving**
Calories: 315; Total Fat: 24g; Carbs: 12g; Net Carbs: 5g; Fiber: 7g; Protein: 16g

1. Preheat the oven to 425°F. Line a baking sheet with aluminum foil or a silicone baking mat.

2. Rub the tilapia with the olive oil, and then coat it with 2 teaspoons of Tajín seasoning salt. Place the fish in the prepared pan.

3. Bake for 15 minutes, or until the fish is opaque when you pierce it with a fork. Put the fish on a cooling rack and let it sit for 4 minutes.

4. Meanwhile, in a medium bowl, gently mix to combine the coleslaw and the mayo sauce. You don't want the cabbage super wet, just enough to dress it. Add the mashed avocado and the remaining 2 teaspoons of Tajín seasoning salt to the coleslaw, and season with pink Himalayan salt and pepper. Divide the salad between two bowls.

5. Use two forks to shred the fish into small pieces, and add it to the bowls.

6. Top the fish with a drizzle of mayo sauce and serve.

*INGREDIENT TIP* If you don't have Spicy Red Pepper Miso Mayo, the Avocado-Lime Crema (page 168) will also work nicely.

# SCALLOPS WITH CREAMY BACON SAUCE

I love big, juicy scallops cooked just right and drenched in a creamy sauce. When looking for them, choose sea scallops, which are much larger than bay scallops, and avoid frozen scallops, which are harder to work with. Don't forget to remove the small side muscle from the sea scallops before rinsing.

**30-MINUTE**

**SERVES 2**
**PREP** 5 minutes
**COOK** 20 minutes

4 bacon slices

1 cup heavy (whipping) cream

1 tablespoon butter

¼ cup grated Parmesan cheese

Pink Himalayan salt

Freshly ground black pepper

1 tablespoon ghee

8 large sea scallops, rinsed and patted dry

**Per Batch**
Calories: 1563; Total Fat: 145g; Carbs: 21g; Net Carbs: 20g; Fiber: 1g; Protein: 47g

**Per Serving**
Calories: 782; Total Fat: 73g; Carbs: 11g; Net Carbs: 10g; Fiber: 0g; Protein: 24g

1. In a medium skillet over medium-high heat, cook the bacon on both sides until crispy, about 8 minutes. Transfer the bacon to a paper towel–lined plate.

2. Lower the heat to medium. Add the cream, butter, and Parmesan cheese to the bacon grease, and season with a pinch of pink Himalayan salt and pepper. Reduce the heat to low and cook, stirring constantly, until the sauce thickens and is reduced by 50 percent, about 10 minutes.

3. In a separate large skillet over medium-high heat, heat the ghee until sizzling.

4. Season the scallops with pink Himalayan salt and pepper, and add them to the skillet. Cook for just 1 minute per side. Do not crowd the scallops; if your pan isn't large enough, cook them in two batches. You want the scallops golden on each side.

5. Transfer the scallops to a paper towel–lined plate.

6. Divide the cream sauce between two plates, crumble the bacon on top of the cream sauce, and top with 4 scallops each. Serve immediately.

## VARIATIONS

This recipe is very rich, so fresh flavors make perfect additions:

- Toss 6 ounces of fresh spinach in a small skillet with 1 tablespoon of butter over medium-high heat. Cook just until wilted, about 1 minute. Fold into the cream sauce just before serving the scallop dish.
- Squeeze the juice from ½ lemon, and stir it into the cream sauce before serving. Garnish the scallops with 1 tablespoon of chopped fresh Italian parsley.

# SHRIMP AND AVOCADO LETTUCE CUPS

Lettuce cups are such a great alternative to salad, and more fun to eat. You want to pick the largest butter lettuce leaves and fill them to the brim with yummy shrimp, creamy avocado, and juicy tomatoes. The Spicy Red Pepper Miso Mayo is a condiment I really love—a zesty vegan mayo that adds a tasty kick to every food.

**30-MINUTE**
**ONE PAN**

**SERVES 2**
**PREP** 10 minutes
**COOK** 5 minutes

1 tablespoon ghee

½ pound shrimp (I use defrosted Trader Joe's Frozen Medium Cooked Shrimp, which are peeled and deveined, with tail off)

½ cup halved grape tomatoes

½ avocado, sliced

Pink Himalayan salt

Freshly ground black pepper

4 butter lettuce leaves, rinsed and patted dry

1 tablespoon Spicy Red Pepper Miso Mayo

**Per Batch**
Calories: 652; Total Fat: 36g; Carbs: 14g; Net Carbs: 8g; Fiber: 6g; Protein: 66g

**Per Serving**
Calories: 326; Total Fat: 11g; Carbs: 7g; Net Carbs: 4g; Fiber: 3g; Protein: 33g

1. In a medium skillet over medium-high heat, heat the ghee. Add the shrimp and cook. (I use cooked shrimp, so they take only about 1 minute to heat through, and I flip them halfway through cooking. Uncooked shrimp take about 2 minutes to cook.) Season with pink Himalayan salt and pepper. Shrimp are cooked when they turn pink and opaque.

2. Season the tomatoes and avocado with pink Himalayan salt and pepper.

3. Divide the lettuce cups between two plates. Fill each cup with shrimp, tomatoes, and avocado. Drizzle the mayo sauce on top and serve.

*SUBSTITUTION TIP* Spicy Red Pepper Miso Mayo is available in most supermarkets. But if you can't find it, you can make your own Sriracha Mayo (page 170).

# GARLIC BUTTER SHRIMP

You only have to wait 15 minutes to get this buttery goodness into your mouth! I love a meal that can be made all in one pan, and I love a meal where butter is one of the main ingredients, so this is a perfect meal for me and for anyone on the keto diet.

**30-MINUTE**
**ONE PAN**

**SERVES 2**
**PREP** 10 minutes
**COOK** 15 minutes

3 tablespoons butter

½ pound shrimp (I use defrosted Trader Joe's Frozen Medium Cooked Shrimp, which are peeled and deveined, with tail off)

Pink Himalayan salt

Freshly ground black pepper

1 lemon, halved

2 garlic cloves, crushed

¼ teaspoon red pepper flakes (optional)

**Per Batch**
Calories: 658; Total Fat: 40g; Carbs: 10g; Net Carbs: 8g; Fiber: 2g; Protein: 64g

**Per Serving**
Calories: 329; Total Fat: 20g; Carbs: 5g; Net Carbs: 4g; Fiber: 1g; Protein: 32g

1. Preheat the oven to 425°F.

2. Place the butter in an 8-inch baking dish, and pop it into the oven while it is preheating, just until the butter melts.

3. Sprinkle the shrimp with pink Himalayan salt and pepper.

4. Slice one half of the lemon in thin slices, and cut the other half into 2 wedges.

5. In the baking dish, add the shrimp and garlic to the butter. The shrimp should be in a single layer. Add the lemon slices. Sprinkle the top of the fish with the red pepper flakes (if using).

6. Bake the shrimp for 15 minutes, stirring halfway through.

7. Remove the shrimp from the oven, and squeeze juice from the 2 lemon wedges over the dish. Serve hot.

*INGREDIENT TIP* Use the extra butter sauce to pour over zoodles or Miracle Noodles, to serve alongside the shrimp.

# PARMESAN-GARLIC SALMON WITH ASPARAGUS

This is a go-to meal for me. I use either individual fillets of salmon or one large fillet. The delicious garlic-butter sauce covers the salmon and asparagus, creating wonderful flavor.

30-MINUTE
ONE PAN

**SERVES 2**
**PREP** 10 minutes
**COOK** 15 minutes

2 (6-ounce) salmon
fillets, skin on

Pink Himalayan salt

Freshly ground
black pepper

1 pound fresh asparagus,
ends snapped off

3 tablespoons butter

2 garlic cloves, minced

¼ cup grated
Parmesan cheese

**Per Batch**
Calories: 867; Total Fat: 52g;
Carbs: 20g; Net Carbs: 11g;
Fiber: 10g; Protein: 83g

**Per Serving**
Calories: 434; Total Fat: 26g;
Carbs: 10g; Net Carbs: 6g;
Fiber: 5g; Protein: 42g

1. Preheat the oven to 400°F. Line a baking sheet with aluminum foil or a silicone baking mat.

2. Pat the salmon dry with a paper towel, and season both sides with pink Himalayan salt and pepper.

3. Place the salmon in the middle of the prepared pan, and arrange the asparagus around the salmon.

4. In a small saucepan over medium heat, melt the butter. Add the minced garlic and stir until the garlic just begins to brown, about 3 minutes.

5. Drizzle the garlic-butter sauce over the salmon and asparagus, and top both with the Parmesan cheese.

6. Bake until the salmon is cooked and the asparagus is crisp-tender, about 12 minutes. You can switch the oven to broil at the end of cooking time for about 3 minutes to get a nice char on the asparagus.

7. Serve hot.

*SUBSTITUTION TIP* If you don't have asparagus, you could use fresh green beans.

# SEARED-SALMON SHIRATAKI RICE BOWLS

I love poke bowls. I have them all the time because raw salmon is one of my favorite foods. I may not be able to technically call this creation "poke," but it was inspired by the same flavors.

**SERVES 2**
**PREP** 10 minutes,
plus 30 minutes to marinate
**COOK** 10 minutes

2 (6-ounce) salmon
fillets, skin on

4 tablespoons soy sauce (or
coconut aminos), divided

2 small Persian cucumbers
or ½ large English
cucumber

1 tablespoon ghee

1 (8-ounce) pack
Miracle Shirataki Rice

1 avocado, diced

Pink Himalayan salt

Freshly ground
black pepper

**Per Batch**
Calories: 655; Total Fat: 35g;
Carbs: 15g; Net Carbs: 9g;
Fiber: 6g; Protein: 71g

**Per Serving**
Calories: 328; Total Fat: 18g;
Carbs: 8g; Net Carbs: 5g;
Fiber: 3g; Protein: 36g

1. Place the salmon in an 8-inch baking dish, and add 3 tablespoons of soy sauce. Cover and marinate in the refrigerator for 30 minutes.

2. Meanwhile, slice the cucumbers thin, put them in a small bowl, and add the remaining 1 tablespoon of soy sauce. Set aside to marinate.

3. In a medium skillet over medium heat, melt the ghee. Add the salmon fillets skin-side down. Pour some of the soy sauce marinade over the salmon, and sear the fish for 3 to 4 minutes on each side.

4. Meanwhile, in a large saucepan, cook the shirataki rice per package instructions:

    1. Rinse the shirataki rice in cold water in a colander.

    2. In a saucepan filled with boiling water, cook the rice for 2 minutes.

    3. Pour the rice into the colander. Dry out the pan.

    4. Transfer the rice to the dry pan and dry roast over medium heat until dry and opaque.

5. Season the avocado with pink Himalayan salt and pepper.

6. Place the salmon fillets on a plate, and remove the skin.
Cut the salmon into bite-size pieces.

7. Assemble the rice bowls: In two bowls, make a layer of the
cooked Miracle Rice. Top each with the cucumbers, avocado,
and salmon, and serve.

**VARIATIONS**

The fun part of poke bowls is customizing the toppings!
Some of my favorites include:

- Miso Mayo
- Furikake (sesame seed and seaweed mixture)
- Fresh cooked crab
- Sliced scallions
- Fresh sliced, peeled ginger
- Wasabi

# PORK RIND SALMON CAKES

This fish-cake recipe is easy to make because it uses canned salmon. I love Wild Planet's canned salmon because it is fresh-caught wild pink salmon. The taste is amazing, and I enjoy knowing I am eating the highest-quality product. The crushed pork rinds help hold the cakes together, like a bread-crumb crust but with more flavor.

**30-MINUTE**

**SERVES 2**
**PREP** 10 minutes
**COOK** 10 minutes

6 ounces canned Alaska wild salmon, drained

2 tablespoons crushed pork rinds

1 egg, lightly beaten

3 tablespoons mayonnaise, divided

Pink Himalayan salt

Freshly ground black pepper

1 tablespoon ghee

½ tablespoon Dijon mustard

**Per Batch**
Calories: 724; Total Fat: 61g;
Carbs: 2g; Net Carbs: 2g;
Fiber: 0g; Protein: 47g

**Per Serving**
Calories: 362; Total Fat: 31g;
Carbs: 1g; Net Carbs: 1g;
Fiber: 0g; Protein: 24g

1. In a medium bowl, mix to combine the salmon, pork rinds, egg, and 1½ tablespoons of mayonnaise, and season with pink Himalayan salt and pepper.

2. With the salmon mixture, form patties the size of hockey pucks or smaller. Keep patting the patties until they keep together.

3. In a medium skillet over medium-high heat, melt the ghee. When the ghee sizzles, place the salmon patties in the pan. Cook for about 3 minutes per side, until browned. Transfer the patties to a paper towel–lined plate.

4. In a small bowl, mix together the remaining 1½ tablespoons of mayonnaise and the mustard.

5. Serve the salmon cakes with the mayo-mustard dipping sauce.

*INGREDIENT TIP*  I recommend purchasing wild-caught salmon versus farmed. Some stores will carry both, and from my experience, if it is labeled "Atlantic salmon," it is farmed, so make sure you read the labels.

# CREAMY DILL SALMON

Salmon is my favorite food. I enjoy it in all forms: smoked, baked, or seared. This salmon recipe is so easy and so creamy that I love to make it for guests. Mayonnaise is a delicious way to create incredibly juicy fish or poultry and to get some healthy fats. And the fresh dill is the perfect herbal accent for salmon.

**30-MINUTE**
**ONE PAN**

**SERVES 2**
**PREP** 10 minutes
**COOK** 10 minutes

2 tablespoons ghee, melted

2 (6-ounce) salmon
fillets, skin on

Pink Himalayan salt

Freshly ground
black pepper

¼ cup mayonnaise

1 tablespoon Dijon mustard

2 tablespoons minced
fresh dill

Pinch garlic powder

**Per Batch**
Calories: 1019; Total Fat: 82g;
Carbs: 4g; Net Carbs: 3g;
Fiber: 1g; Protein: 66g

**Per Serving**
Calories: 510; Total Fat: 41g;
Carbs: 2g; Net Carbs: 2g;
Fiber: 1g; Protein: 33g

1. Preheat the oven to 450°F. Coat a 9-by-13-inch baking dish with the ghee.

2. Pat dry the salmon with paper towels, season on both sides with pink Himalayan salt and pepper, and place in the prepared baking dish.

3. In a small bowl, mix to combine the mayonnaise, mustard, dill, and garlic powder.

4. Slather the mayonnaise sauce on top of both salmon fillets so that it fully covers the tops.

5. Bake for 7 to 9 minutes, depending on how you like your salmon—7 minutes for medium-rare and 9 minutes for well-done—and serve.

*INGREDIENT TIP* A lot of people might be unsure about eating the skin of the salmon, but a large amount of the healthy fats in salmon is found in the skin. Also, cooking the fish with the skin on helps retain moisture while cooking.

# CHICKEN-BASIL ALFREDO WITH SHIRATAKI NOODLES

Miracle Noodles are one of my favorite products, which I discovered after going keto. At first you might find them puzzling, because the cooking process for these noodles is different from what you are used to. But they can totally satisfy that pasta craving. This decadent "pasta" dish uses shirataki noodles, creamy Alfredo sauce, chicken, and fresh herbs. It is so filling and delicious!

**30-MINUTE**

**SERVES 2**
**PREP** 10 minutes
**COOK** 15 minutes

**FOR THE NOODLES**
1 (7-ounce) package Miracle Noodle Fettuccini Shirataki Noodles

**FOR THE SAUCE**
1 tablespoon olive oil

4 ounces cooked shredded chicken (I usually use a store-bought rotisserie chicken)

Pink Himalayan salt

Freshly ground black pepper

1 cup Alfredo Sauce (page 175), or any brand you like

¼ cup grated Parmesan cheese

2 tablespoons chopped fresh basil leaves

**Per Batch**
Calories: 1346; Total Fat: 122g; Carbs: 8g; Net Carbs: 8g; Fiber: 0g; Protein: 58g

**Per Serving**
Calories: 673; Total Fat: 61g; Carbs: 4g; Net Carbs: 4g; Fiber: 0g; Protein: 29g

**TO MAKE THE NOODLES**

Follow the instructions on the package:

1. In a colander, rinse the noodles with cold water (shirataki noodles naturally have a smell, and rinsing with cold water will help remove this).

2. Fill a large saucepan with water and bring to a boil over high heat. Add the noodles and boil for 2 minutes. Drain.

3. Transfer the noodles to a large, dry skillet over medium-low heat to evaporate any moisture. Do not grease the skillet; it must be dry. Transfer the noodles to a plate and set aside.

**TO MAKE THE SAUCE**

1. In the saucepan over medium heat, heat the olive oil. Add the cooked chicken. Season with pink Himalayan salt and pepper.

2. Pour the Alfredo sauce over the chicken, and cook until warm. Season with more pink Himalayan salt and pepper.

3. Add the dried noodles to the sauce mixture, and toss until combined.

4. Divide the pasta between two plates, top each with the Parmesan cheese and chopped basil, and serve.

*SUBSTITUTION TIP* To make this meal vegetarian, you need only replace the shredded chicken with sautéed mushrooms.

# CHICKEN QUESADILLA

There is something so simple and satisfying about a chicken quesadilla. It is one of those universally loved dishes. I make them often for my daughter because most of the time, if you ask her what she wants, this is what she requests. There are a lot of low-carb tortilla options on the market now, which makes it easier than ever to enjoy a quesadilla without taking in lots of carbs.

**30-MINUTE**
**ONE PAN**

**SERVES 2**
**PREP** 5 minutes
**COOK** 5 minutes

1 tablespoon olive oil

2 low-carbohydrate tortillas

½ cup shredded Mexican blend cheese

2 ounces shredded chicken (I usually use a store-bought rotisserie chicken)

1 teaspoon Tajín seasoning salt

2 tablespoons sour cream

**Per Batch**
Calories: 827; Total Fat: 55g;
Carbs: 48g; Net Carbs: 14g
Fiber: 34g; Protein: 52g

**Per Serving**
Calories: 414; Total Fat: 28g;
Carbs: 24g; Net Carbs: 7g
Fiber: 17g; Protein: 26g

1. In a large skillet over medium-high heat, heat the olive oil. Add a tortilla, then layer on top ¼ cup of cheese, the chicken, the Tajín seasoning, and the remaining ¼ cup of cheese. Top with the second tortilla.

2. Peek under the edge of the bottom tortilla to monitor how it is browning. Once the bottom tortilla gets golden and the cheese begins to melt, after about 2 minutes, flip the quesadilla over. The second side will cook faster, about 1 minute.

3. Once the second tortilla is crispy and golden, transfer the quesadilla to a cutting board and let sit for 2 minutes. Cut the quesadilla into 4 wedges using a pizza cutter or chef's knife.

4. Transfer half the quesadilla to each of two plates. Add 1 tablespoon of sour cream to each plate, and serve hot.

*INGREDIENT TIP* The olive oil in the skillet is what makes the tortilla beautifully golden and crispy.

**VARIATIONS**
You can add nearly endless numbers of tasty elements to a quesadilla. Try traditional Mexican inclusions or unexpected combinations:

- Leftover sliced steak and avocado slices are delicious fillings.
- For an Italian take on a quesadilla, try shredded mozzarella, pepperoni, sliced pepperoncini, and grated Parmesan.

# GARLIC-PARMESAN CHICKEN WINGS

I love making these slow-cooker chicken wings. I always start them on a weekend morning, and they just fill the house with amazing butter and garlic fragrances all day. Then, at the very end of the cooking time, I pop them under the broiler to get them to crispy perfection.

**SERVES 2**
**PREP** 10 minutes
**COOK** 3 hours

8 tablespoons
(1 stick) butter

2 garlic cloves, minced

1 tablespoon dried Italian seasoning

¼ cup grated Parmesan cheese, plus ½ cup

Pink Himalayan salt

Freshly ground
black pepper

1 pound chicken wings

**Per Batch**
Calories: 1476; Total Fat: 131g;
Carbs: 7g; Net Carbs: 7g;
Fiber: 0g; Protein: 77g

**Per Serving**
Calories: 738; Total Fat: 66g;
Carbs: 4g; Net Carbs: 4g;
Fiber: 0g; Protein: 39g

1. With the crock insert in place, preheat the slow cooker to high. Line a baking sheet with aluminum foil or a silicone baking mat.

2. Put the butter, garlic, Italian seasoning, and ¼ cup of Parmesan cheese in the slow cooker, and season with pink Himalayan salt and pepper. Allow the butter to melt, and stir the ingredients until well mixed.

3. Add the chicken wings and stir until coated with the butter mixture.

4. Cover the slow cooker and cook for 2 hours and 45 minutes.

5. Preheat the broiler.

6. Transfer the wings to the prepared baking sheet, sprinkle the remaining ½ cup of Parmesan cheese over the wings, and cook under the broiler until crispy, about 5 minutes.

7. Serve hot.

*INGREDIENT TIP* I like to buy a combination of fresh (not frozen) chicken wingettes and drummettes.

# CHICKEN SKEWERS WITH PEANUT SAUCE

A traditional chicken satay would generally have a lot more ingredients than this recipe, so I am not calling it a satay, although this recipe was inspired by those flavors. I rarely eat peanut butter, but I can't pass up a spicy peanut sauce! Add as much or as little Sriracha sauce as you want to control the spice level.

**SERVES 2**
**PREP** 10 minutes, plus 1 hour to marinate
**COOK** 15 minutes

1 pound boneless skinless chicken breast, cut into chunks

3 tablespoons soy sauce (or coconut aminos), divided

½ teaspoon Sriracha sauce, plus ¼ teaspoon

3 teaspoons toasted sesame oil, divided

Ghee, for oiling

2 tablespoons peanut butter

Pink Himalayan salt

Freshly ground black pepper

**Per Batch**
Calories: 1171; Total Fat: 57g; Carbs: 11g; Net Carbs: 9g; Fiber: 2g; Protein: 149g

**Per Serving**
Calories: 586; Total Fat: 29g; Carbs: 6g; Net Carbs: 5g; Fiber: 1g; Protein: 75g

1. In a large zip-top bag, combine the chicken chunks with 2 tablespoons of soy sauce, ½ teaspoon of Sriracha sauce, and 2 teaspoons of sesame oil. Seal the bag, and let the chicken marinate for an hour or so in the refrigerator or up to overnight.

2. If you are using wood 8-inch skewers, soak them in water for 30 minutes before using.

3. I like to use my grill pan for the skewers, because I don't have an outdoor grill. If you don't have a grill pan, you can use a large skillet. Preheat your grill pan or grill to low. Oil the grill pan with ghee.

4. Thread the chicken chunks onto the skewers.

5. Cook the skewers over low heat for 10 to 15 minutes, flipping halfway through.

6. Meanwhile, mix the peanut dipping sauce. Stir together the remaining 1 tablespoon of soy sauce, ¼ teaspoon of Sriracha sauce, 1 teaspoon of sesame oil, and the peanut butter. Season with pink Himalayan salt and pepper.

7. Serve the chicken skewers with a small dish of the peanut sauce.

*INGREDIENT TIP* Coconut aminos tastes just like soy sauce but is gluten-free and Paleo-friendly.

# BRAISED CHICKEN THIGHS WITH KALAMATA OLIVES

Chicken thighs are not something I had ever made until the past couple of years. My daughter loves them, and I love them, too, because they are so tender and tasty, with crispy skin—but they take a little practice to get right. The key is starting them on the stove top, leaving them alone so the skin can get nice and crispy, and then transferring them to the oven to finish cooking and get tender. Use a cast iron skillet or other oven-safe pan.

ONE PAN

**SERVES 2**
**PREP** 10 minutes
**COOK** 40 minutes

4 chicken thighs, skin on

Pink Himalayan salt

Freshly ground
black pepper

2 tablespoons ghee

½ cup chicken broth

1 lemon, ½ sliced and
½ juiced

½ cup pitted
Kalamata olives

2 tablespoons butter

**Per Batch**
Calories: 1134; Total Fat: 94g;
Carbs: 4g; Net Carbs: 4g;
Fiber: 3g; Protein: 65g

**Per Serving**
Calories: 567; Total Fat: 47g;
Carbs: 4g; Net Carbs: 2g;
Fiber: 2g; Protein: 33g

1. Preheat the oven to 375°F.

2. Pat the chicken thighs dry with paper towels, and season with pink Himalayan salt and pepper.

3. In a medium oven-safe skillet or high-sided baking dish over medium-high heat, melt the ghee. When the ghee has melted and is hot, add the chicken thighs, skin-side down, and leave them for about 8 minutes, or until the skin is brown and crispy.

4. Flip the chicken and cook for 2 minutes on the second side. Around the chicken thighs, pour in the chicken broth, and add the lemon slices, lemon juice, and olives.

5. Bake in the oven for about 30 minutes, until the chicken is cooked through.

6. Add the butter to the broth mixture.

7. Divide the chicken and olives between two plates and serve.

*INGREDIENT TIP* You can use any of your favorite olives in this dish instead of Kalamata if you like.

# BUTTERY GARLIC CHICKEN

Chicken drenched in butter? Sign me up! This chicken is so moist and delicious, and you will definitely want to spoon all of the excess butter over the top at the end.

**SERVES 2**
**PREP** 5 minutes
**COOK** 40 minutes

2 tablespoons ghee, melted

2 boneless skinless chicken breasts

Pink Himalayan salt

Freshly ground black pepper

1 tablespoon dried Italian seasoning

4 tablespoons butter

2 garlic cloves, minced

¼ cup grated Parmesan cheese

**Per Batch**
Calories: 1283; Total Fat: 89g; Carbs: 3g; Net Carbs: 3g; Fiber: 0g; Protein: 114g

**Per Serving**
Calories: 642; Total Fat: 45g; Carbs: 2g; Net Carbs: 2g; Fiber: 0g; Protein: 57g

1. Preheat the oven to 375°F. Choose a baking dish that is large enough to hold both chicken breasts and coat it with the ghee.

2. Pat dry the chicken breasts and season with pink Himalayan salt, pepper, and Italian seasoning. Place the chicken in the baking dish.

3. In a medium skillet over medium heat, melt the butter. Add the minced garlic, and cook for about 5 minutes. You want the garlic very lightly browned but not burned.

4. Remove the butter-garlic mixture from the heat, and pour it over the chicken breasts.

5. Roast the chicken in the oven for 30 to 35 minutes, until cooked through. Sprinkle some of the Parmesan cheese on top of each chicken breast. Let the chicken rest in the baking dish for 5 minutes.

6. Divide the chicken between two plates, spoon the butter sauce over the chicken, and serve.

*SUBSTITUTION TIP* If you don't have dried Italian seasoning, you can make your own mix from dried herbs and spices you may have in your cupboard. Mix together as many of these ingredients as you have: 1 teaspoon each of dried basil, oregano, thyme, rosemary, sage, garlic powder, and cilantro.

# CHEESY BACON AND BROCCOLI CHICKEN

I think I would like anything smothered in cream cheese and topped with bacon, and this meal is no exception. This recipe gives you instructions for baking the chicken breast and bacon, but I typically make this dish when I have leftovers of both items so I can put this together super fast.

**SERVES 2**
**PREP** 10 minutes
**COOK** 1 hour

2 tablespoons ghee

2 boneless skinless chicken breasts

Pink Himalayan salt

Freshly ground black pepper

4 bacon slices

6 ounces cream cheese, at room temperature

2 cups frozen broccoli florets, thawed

½ cup shredded Cheddar cheese

**Per Batch**
Calories: 1869; Total Fat: 132g; Carbs: 20g; Net Carbs: 15g; Fiber: 5g; Protein: 149g

**Per Serving**
Calories: 935; Total Fat: 66g; Carbs: 10g; Net Carbs: 8g; Fiber: 3g; Protein: 75g

1. Preheat the oven to 375°F.

2. Choose a baking dish that is large enough to hold both chicken breasts and coat it with the ghee.

3. Pat dry the chicken breasts with a paper towel, and season with pink Himalayan salt and pepper.

4. Place the chicken breasts and the bacon slices in the baking dish, and bake for 25 minutes.

5. Transfer the chicken to a cutting board and use two forks to shred it. Season it again with pink Himalayan salt and pepper.

6. Place the bacon on a paper towel–lined plate to crisp up, and then crumble it.

7. In a medium bowl, mix to combine the cream cheese, shredded chicken, broccoli, and half of the bacon crumbles. Transfer the chicken mixture to the baking dish, and top with the Cheddar and the remaining half of the bacon crumbles.

8. Bake until the cheese is bubbling and browned, about 35 minutes, and serve.

*INGREDIENT TIP* You could replace the broccoli with cauliflower if you prefer.

# PARMESAN BAKED CHICKEN

I have been making this chicken dish forever. It is the easiest recipe ever: You basically smother the chicken in mayonnaise, and the mayonnaise makes it tender and juicy. Over the years I have added keto-friendly crushed pork rinds and some Italian seasoning, making this dish perfect for a keto diet.

**30-MINUTE**
**ONE PAN**

**SERVES 2**
**PREP** 5 minutes
**COOK** 20 minutes

2 tablespoons ghee

2 boneless skinless chicken breasts

Pink Himalayan salt

Freshly ground black pepper

½ cup mayonnaise

¼ cup grated Parmesan cheese

1 tablespoon dried Italian seasoning

¼ cup crushed pork rinds

**Per Batch**
Calories: 1700; Total Fat: 133g;
Carbs: 4g; Net Carbs: 4g;
Fiber: 0g; Protein: 119g

**Per Serving**
Calories: 850; Total Fat: 67g;
Carbs: 2g; Net Carbs: 2g;
Fiber: 0g; Protein: 60g

1. Preheat the oven to 425°F. Choose a baking dish that is large enough to hold both chicken breasts and coat it with the ghee.

2. Pat dry the chicken breasts with a paper towel, season with pink Himalayan salt and pepper, and place in the prepared baking dish.

3. In a small bowl, mix to combine the mayonnaise, Parmesan cheese, and Italian seasoning.

4. Slather the mayonnaise mixture evenly over the chicken breasts, and sprinkle the crushed pork rinds on top of the mayonnaise mixture.

5. Bake until the topping is browned, about 20 minutes, and serve.

*INGREDIENT TIP* You can leave out the pork rinds if you don't have them in your pantry, but they add a nice texture.

# CRUNCHY CHICKEN MILANESE

When in doubt, I make this chicken dish. I love it, my daughter loves it—in fact, I can't imagine anyone not liking it. The key to the dish is pounding the chicken thin so that it cooks quickly.

**30-MINUTE**

**SERVES 2**
**PREP** 10 minutes
**COOK** 10 minutes

2 boneless skinless chicken breasts

½ cup coconut flour

1 teaspoon ground cayenne pepper

Pink Himalayan salt

Freshly ground black pepper

1 egg, lightly beaten

½ cup crushed pork rinds

2 tablespoons olive oil

**Per Batch**
Calories: 1207; Total Fat: 57g; Carbs: 33g; Net Carbs: 13g; Fiber: 20g; Protein: 130g

**Per Serving**
Calories: 604; Total Fat: 29g; Carbs: 17g; Net Carbs: 7g; Fiber: 10g; Protein: 65g

1. Pound the chicken breasts with a heavy mallet until they are about ½ inch thick. (If you don't have a kitchen mallet, you can use the thick rim of a heavy plate.)

2. Prepare two separate prep plates and one small, shallow bowl:

   - On plate 1, put the coconut flour, cayenne pepper, pink Himalayan salt, and pepper. Mix together.

   - Crack the egg into the small bowl, and lightly beat it with a fork or whisk.

   - On plate 2, put the crushed pork rinds.

3. In a large skillet over medium-high heat, heat the olive oil.

4. Dredge 1 chicken breast on both sides in the coconut-flour mixture. Dip the chicken into the egg, and coat both sides. Dredge the chicken in the pork-rind mixture, pressing the pork rinds into the chicken so they stick. Place the coated chicken in the hot skillet and repeat with the other chicken breast.

5. Cook the chicken for 3 to 5 minutes on each side, until brown, crispy, and cooked through, and serve.

*SUBSTITUTION TIP* You can replace the cayenne pepper with grated Parmesan cheese if you prefer milder food.

# BAKED GARLIC AND PAPRIKA CHICKEN LEGS

Drumsticks are always worth the wait. I love layering on flavors and getting the chicken skin crispy. The combination of flavors of the garlic, paprika, and herbs will excite your palate.

**SERVES 2**
**PREP** 10 minutes
**COOK** 55 minutes

1 pound chicken drumsticks, skin on

Pink Himalayan salt

Freshly ground black pepper

2 tablespoons ghee

2 garlic cloves, minced

1 teaspoon paprika

1 teaspoon dried Italian seasoning

½ pound fresh green beans

1 tablespoon olive oil

**Per Batch**
Calories: 1400; Total Fat: 90g;
Carbs: 19g; Net Carbs: 12g;
Fiber: 7g; Protein: 126g

**Per Serving**
Calories: 700; Total Fat: 45g;
Carbs: 10g; Net Carbs: 6g;
Fiber: 4g; Protein: 63g

1. Preheat the oven to 425°F. Line a 9-by-13-inch baking pan with aluminum foil or a silicone baking mat.

2. Pat the chicken legs dry with paper towels, put them in a large bowl, and apply pink Himalayan salt and pepper all over the skin on both sides.

3. In a small saucepan over medium-low heat, combine the ghee, garlic, paprika, and Italian seasoning. Stir to combine for 30 seconds, and let sit for 5 minutes while the flavors combine.

4. Pour the sauce over the chicken legs, and toss to coat evenly. Season with more pink Himalayan salt and pepper.

5. Arrange the chicken legs on one side of the prepared pan, leaving room for the vegetables later.

6. Bake the chicken for 30 minutes, then remove the pan from the oven. Spread the green beans over the empty half of the pan, and turn the chicken legs. Drizzle the beans with the olive oil, and season with pink Himalayan salt and pepper.

7. Roast for 15 to 20 minutes more, until the chicken is cooked through and the skin is crispy, and serve.

*SUBSTITUTION TIP* You can replace the Italian herbs with any herbs or spices you prefer, such as an Indian spice mix like garam masala, or Chinese five-spice powder.

# CREAMY SLOW-COOKER CHICKEN

A creamy slow cooker meal is perfect for those chilly days. You can make this dish very quickly and then enjoy the aromas for the next 4 hours while it cooks. The fresh spinach added toward the end of the cooking time adds beautiful color and freshness.

**SERVES 2**
**PREP** 10 minutes
**COOK** 4 hours 15 minutes

1 tablespoon ghee

2 boneless skinless chicken breasts

1 cup Alfredo Sauce (page 175), or any brand you like

¼ cup chopped sun-dried tomatoes

¼ cup grated Parmesan cheese

Pink Himalayan salt

Freshly ground black pepper

2 cups fresh spinach

**Per Batch**
Calories: 1800; Total Fat: 131g; Carbs: 17g; Net Carbs: 14g; Fiber: 3g; Protein: 139g

**Per Serving**
Calories: 900; Total Fat: 66g; Carbs: 9g; Net Carbs: 7g; Fiber: 2g; Protein: 70g

1. In a medium skillet over medium-high heat, melt the ghee. Add the chicken and cook, about 4 minutes on each side, until brown.

2. With the crock insert in place, transfer the chicken to the slow cooker. Set the slow cooker to low.

3. In a small bowl, mix to combine the Alfredo sauce, sun-dried tomatoes, and Parmesan cheese, and season with pink Himalayan salt and pepper. Pour the sauce over the chicken.

4. Cover and cook on low for 4 hours, or until the chicken is cooked through.

5. Add the fresh spinach. Cover and cook for 5 minutes more, until the spinach is slightly wilted, and serve.

*SUBSTITUTION TIP* You can replace the chicken with pork chops and follow the same instructions.

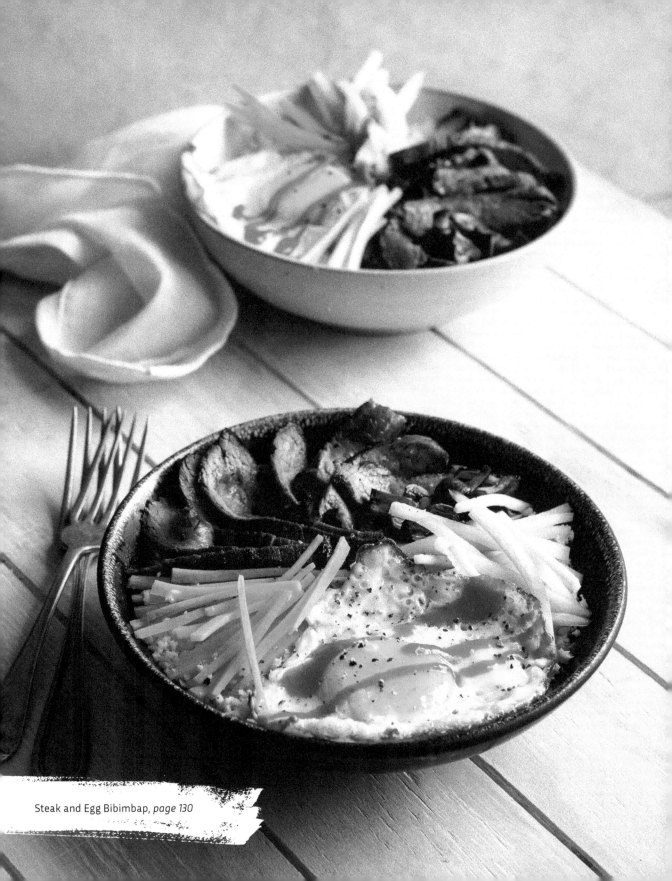

Steak and Egg Bibimbap, *page 130*

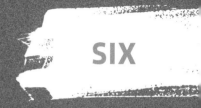

# SIX

# PORK & BEEF ENTRÉES

When people think of the keto diet, pork and beef are definitely two of the most enjoyed foods that come to mind. This chapter offers dishes that are simple and packed with flavor. From slow-cooker meals that you can let cook all day to dishes that are ready in less than 30 minutes, this chapter's variety is tasty and satisfying.

# BLTA CUPS

What's better than a cup made of bacon? In my opinion, you can pair almost anything with bacon, but a classic is bacon paired with lettuce, tomato, and avocado. You'll love these bacon cups, which are full of flavor.

ONE PAN

**SERVES 2**
**PREP** 5 minutes
**COOK** 20 minutes, plus
10 minutes to rest

12 bacon slices

¼ head romaine lettuce, chopped

½ avocado, diced

½ cup halved grape tomatoes

2 tablespoons sour cream

**Per Batch**
Calories: 708; Total Fat: 56g;
Carbs: 13g; Net Carbs: 6g;
Fiber: 7g; Protein: 39g

**Per Serving** (2 bowls)
Calories: 354; Total Fat: 28g;
Carbs: 6.5g; Net Carbs: 3g;
Fiber: 3.5g; Protein: 19.5g

1. Preheat the oven to 400°F. You will need a muffin tin. (I use a jumbo muffin tin, but you can use a standard muffin tin if that's what you have.)

2. Turn a muffin tin upside down, and lay it on a baking sheet. Make a cross with 2 bacon strip halves over the upside-down muffin tin. Take 2 more bacon strip halves and put them around the perimeter of the crossed halves. Take 1 full bacon strip and circle it around the base of the upside down tin and then use a toothpick to hold that piece together tightly. Repeat to make 4 cups total.

3. Bake for 20 minutes, or until the bacon is crispy. Transfer to a cooling rack and let rest for at least 10 minutes.

4. Once the bacon cups have become firm, carefully remove them from the muffin cups and place two cups on each of two plates. Fill the cups evenly with the romaine, add the avocado, tomatoes, and a dollop of sour cream, and serve.

*INGREDIENT TIP* The bacon cups will store well covered in the refrigerator for up to 3 days, so you might want to make extra!

# BUTTER AND HERB PORK CHOPS

Sometimes the simplest flavors are the most delicious. It is hard to go wrong with herbs, butter, and olive oil. The flavors complement the pork beautifully, and the dish bakes quickly so it can go from the kitchen to the dinner table in no more than 30 minutes.

**30-MINUTE**
**ONE PAN**

**SERVES 2**
**PREP** 5 minutes
**COOK** 25 minutes

1 tablespoon butter, plus more for coating

2 boneless pork chops

Pink Himalayan salt

Freshly ground black pepper

1 tablespoon dried Italian seasoning

1 tablespoon chopped fresh flat-leaf Italian parsley

1 tablespoon olive oil

**Per Batch**
Calories: 666; Total Fat: 45g; Carbs: 0g; Net Carbs: 0g; Fiber: 0g; Protein: 62g

**Per Serving**
Calories: 333; Total Fat: 23g; Carbs: 0g; Net Carbs: 0g; Fiber: 0g; Protein: 31g

1. Preheat the oven to 350°F. Choose a baking dish that will hold both pork chops and coat it with the butter.

2. Pat the pork chops dry with a paper towel, place them in the prepared baking dish, and season with pink Himalayan salt, pepper, and Italian seasoning.

3. Top with the fresh parsley, drizzle the olive oil over both pork chops, and top each chop with ½ tablespoon of butter.

4. Bake for 20 to 25 minutes. (Thinner pork chops will cook faster than thicker ones.)

5. Place the pork chops on two plates, spoon the buttery juices over the meat, and serve hot.

*SERVING TIP* This dish is particularly delicious with mashed cauliflower.

# PARMESAN PORK CHOPS AND ROASTED ASPARAGUS

This recipe is perfect for a weeknight meal since everything cooks on one pan. You'll love these, especially their crispy pork rind and Parmesan "breading." The roasted asparagus also contributes some crunchy goodness.

ONE PAN

**SERVES 2**
**PREP** 10 minutes
**COOK** 25 minutes

¼ cup grated
Parmesan cheese

¼ cup crushed pork rinds

1 teaspoon garlic powder

2 boneless pork chops

Pink Himalayan salt

Freshly ground
black pepper

Olive oil, for drizzling

½ pound asparagus spears,
tough ends snapped off

**Per Batch**
Calories: 740; Total Fat: 42g;
Carbs: 12g; Net Carbs: 7g;
Fiber: 5g; Protein: 79g

**Per Serving**
Calories: 370; Total Fat: 21g;
Carbs: 6g; Net Carbs: 4g;
Fiber: 3g; Protein: 40g

1. Preheat the oven to 350°F. Line a baking sheet with aluminum foil or a silicone baking mat.

2. In a medium bowl, mix to combine the Parmesan cheese, pork rinds, and garlic powder.

3. Pat the pork chops dry with a paper towel, and season with pink Himalayan salt and pepper.

4. Place a pork chop in the bowl with the Parmesan–pork rind mixture, and press the "breading" to the pork chop so it sticks. Place the coated pork chop on the prepared baking sheet. Repeat for the second pork chop.

5. Drizzle a small amount of olive oil over each pork chop.

6. Place the asparagus on the baking sheet around the pork chops. Drizzle with olive oil, and season with pink Himalayan salt and pepper. Sprinkle any leftover Parmesan cheese–pork rind mixture over the asparagus.

7. Bake for 20 to 25 minutes. Thinner pork chops will cook faster than thicker ones.

8. Serve hot.

*INGREDIENT TIP* There are a lot of different flavors of pork rinds available now. Feel free to use any of them to add a unique flavor profile to this dish.

# SESAME PORK AND GREEN BEANS

This dinner is quick and flavorful. It celebrates Asian flavors in a healthy and hearty dish that you can create in just minutes on a busy night.

**30-MINUTE**

**SERVES 2**
**PREP** 5 minutes
**COOK** 10 minutes

2 boneless pork chops

Pink Himalayan salt

Freshly ground
black pepper

2 tablespoons toasted
sesame oil, divided

2 tablespoons soy sauce

1 teaspoon Sriracha sauce

1 cup fresh green beans

**Per Batch**
Calories: 732; Total Fat: 48g;
Carbs: 9g; Net Carbs: 6g;
Fiber: 3g; Protein: 65g

**Per Serving**
Calories: 366; Total Fat: 24g;
Carbs: 5g; Net Carbs: 3g;
Fiber: 2g; Protein: 33g

1. On a cutting board, pat the pork chops dry with a paper towel. Slice the chops into strips, and season with pink Himalayan salt and pepper.

2. In a large skillet over medium heat, heat 1 tablespoon of sesame oil.

3. Add the pork strips and cook them for 7 minutes, stirring occasionally.

4. In a small bowl, mix to combine the remaining 1 tablespoon of sesame oil, the soy sauce, and the Sriracha sauce. Pour into the skillet with the pork.

5. Add the green beans to the skillet, reduce the heat to medium-low, and simmer for 3 to 5 minutes.

6. Divide the pork, green beans, and sauce between two wide, shallow bowls and serve.

*SUBSTITUTION TIP* If Sriracha sauce is too spicy for you, you can add peeled, minced fresh ginger instead, which will add flavor and kick but not heat.

# SLOW-COOKER BARBECUE RIBS

Ribs are such a treat. The slow cooker works really well for making ribs. There are many tasty sugar-free barbecue sauces available at the supermarket, making this recipe ever so simple.

ONE POT

**SERVES 2**
**PREP** 10 minutes
**COOK** 4 hours

1 pound pork ribs
Pink Himalayan salt
Freshly ground
black pepper
1 (1.25-ounce) package
dry rib-seasoning rub
½ cup sugar-free
barbecue sauce

**Per Batch**
Calories: 1911; Total Fat: 143g;
Carbs: 10g; Net Carbs: 10g;
Fiber: 0g; Protein: 136g

**Per Serving**
Calories: 956; Total Fat: 72g;
Carbs: 5g; Net Carbs: 5g;
Fiber: 0g; Protein: 68g

1. With the crock insert in place, preheat the slow cooker to high.

2. Generously season the pork ribs with pink Himalayan salt, pepper, and dry rib-seasoning rub.

3. Stand the ribs up along the walls of the slow-cooker insert, with the bonier side facing inward.

4. Pour the barbecue sauce on both sides of the ribs, using just enough to coat.

5. Cover, cook for 4 hours, and serve.

*INGREDIENT TIP* The ribs will be very tender, so be careful removing them from the slow cooker.

# KALUA PORK WITH CABBAGE

My family lived in Honolulu for nine years, and while on the island I fell in love with "plate lunch," and specifically kalua pork. Plate lunch always has a scoop of white rice and macaroni salad, which I have given up for my keto lifestyle, but I can still enjoy kalua pork anytime.

**SERVES 2**
**PREP** 10 minutes
**COOK** 8 hours

1 pound boneless pork butt roast

Pink Himalayan salt

Freshly ground black pepper

1 tablespoon smoked paprika or Liquid Smoke

½ cup water

½ head cabbage, chopped

**Per Batch**
Calories: 1099; Total Fat: 82g; Carbs: 19g; Net Carbs: 10g; Fiber: 9g; Protein: 77g

**Per Serving**
Calories: 550; Total Fat: 41g; Carbs: 10g; Net Carbs: 5g; Fiber: 5g; Protein: 39g

1. With the crock insert in place, preheat the slow cooker to low.

2. Generously season the pork roast with pink Himalayan salt, pepper, and smoked paprika.

3. Place the pork roast in the slow-cooker insert, and add the water.

4. Cover and cook on low for 7 hours.

5. Transfer the cooked pork roast to a plate. Put the chopped cabbage in the bottom of the slow cooker, and put the pork roast back in on top of the cabbage.

6. Cover and cook the cabbage and pork roast for 1 hour.

7. Remove the pork roast from the slow cooker and place it on a baking sheet. Use two forks to shred the pork.

8. Serve the shredded pork hot with the cooked cabbage.

9. Reserve the liquid from the slow cooker to remoisten the pork and cabbage when reheating leftovers.

*SERVING TIP* You can serve the kalua pork alone or over cauliflower rice or enjoy it on a low-carb roll. To make cauliflower rice, simply process cauliflower florets in your food processor or blender to achieve a rice-like consistency. Then sauté the cauliflower rice in olive oil or ghee in a skillet over medium heat for about 5 minutes.

# PORK BURGERS WITH SRIRACHA MAYO

People don't think about ground pork enough when it comes to burgers! Ground pork works beautifully for burgers, and I love adding fresh ingredients to the meat and then topping the dish with a burst of flavor, like that from this Sriracha mayonnaise. Whether you eat your burger with a knife and fork or add lettuce leaves to wrap it up, this is the perfect keto burger.

**30-MINUTE**

**SERVES 2**
**PREP** 10 minutes
**COOK** 10 minutes

12 ounces ground pork

2 scallions, white and green parts, thinly sliced

1 tablespoon toasted sesame oil

Pink Himalayan salt

Freshly ground black pepper

1 tablespoon ghee

1 tablespoon Sriracha sauce

2 tablespoons mayonnaise

**Per Batch**
Calories: 1150; Total Fat: 98g; Carbs: 3g; Net Carbs: 2g; Fiber: 1g; Protein: 62g

**Per Serving**
Calories: 575; Total Fat: 49g; Carbs: 2g; Net Carbs: 1g; Fiber: 1g; Protein: 31g

1. In a large bowl, mix to combine the ground pork with the scallions and sesame oil, and season with pink Himalayan salt and pepper. Form the pork mixture into 2 patties. Create an imprint with your thumb in the middle of each burger so the pork will heat evenly.

2. In a large skillet over medium-high heat, heat the ghee. When the ghee has melted and is very hot, add the burger patties and cook for 4 minutes on each side.

3. Meanwhile, in a small bowl, mix the Sriracha sauce and mayonnaise.

4. Transfer the burgers to a plate and let rest for at least 5 minutes.

5. Top the burgers with the Sriracha mayonnaise and serve.

*INGREDIENT TIP* Sriracha is spicy, so use as little or as much as you want based on your heat tolerance.

# BLUE CHEESE PORK CHOPS

I love this blue cheese sauce. I am convinced you could put it on top of anything and it would be amazing, but I really love it with pork chops. The ingredients of this recipe are perfect for the keto diet, and it's very quick to make.

**30-MINUTE**

**SERVES 2**
**PREP** 5 minutes
**COOK** 10 minutes

2 boneless pork chops

Pink Himalayan salt

Freshly ground
black pepper

2 tablespoons butter

⅓ cup blue cheese crumbles

⅓ cup heavy
(whipping) cream

⅓ cup sour cream

**Per Batch**
Calories: 1338; Total Fat: 109g;
Carbs: 7g; Net Carbs: 7g;
Fiber: 0g; Protein: 81g

**Per Serving**
Calories: 669; Total Fat: 34g;
Carbs: 4g; Net Carbs: 4g;
Fiber: 0g; Protein: 41g

1. Pat the pork chops dry, and season with pink Himalayan salt and pepper.

2. In a medium skillet over medium heat, melt the butter. When the butter melts and is very hot, add the pork chops and sear on each side for 3 minutes.

3. Transfer the pork chops to a plate and let rest for 3 to 5 minutes.

4. In a medium saucepan over medium heat, melt the blue cheese crumbles, stirring frequently so they don't burn.

5. Add the cream and the sour cream to the pan with the blue cheese. Let simmer for a few minutes, stirring occasionally.

6. For an extra kick of flavor in the sauce, pour the pork-chop pan juice into the cheese mixture and stir. Let simmer while the pork chops are resting.

7. Put the pork chops on two plates, pour the blue cheese sauce over the top of each, and serve.

*INGREDIENT TIP* The blue cheese sauce is also delicious poured over vegetables.

# CARNITAS

Carnitas are easy to prep and make ahead for quick meals later in the day. The key is letting the pork cook low and slow and infusing the meat with ingredients like onions and garlic to enhance the flavor of the pork. These are especially tasty in my Carnitas Nachos (page 124).

**SERVES 2**
**PREP** 10 minutes
**COOK** 8 hours

½ tablespoon chili powder

1 tablespoon olive oil

1 pound boneless pork butt roast

2 garlic cloves, minced

½ small onion, diced

Pinch pink Himalayan salt

Pinch freshly ground black pepper

Juice of 1 lime

**Per Batch**
Calories: 892; Total Fat: 51g; Carbs: 12g; Net Carbs: 8g; Fiber: 3g; Protein: 90g

**Per Serving**
Calories: 446; Total Fat: 26g; Carbs: 6g; Net Carbs: 4g; Fiber: 2g; Protein: 45g

1. With the crock insert in place, preheat the slow cooker to low.

2. In a small bowl, mix to combine the chili powder and olive oil, and rub it all over the pork.

3. Place the pork in the slow cooker, fat-side up.

4. Top the pork with the garlic, onion, pink Himalayan salt, pepper, and lime juice.

5. Cover and cook on low for 8 hours.

6. Transfer the pork to a cutting board, shred the meat with two forks, and serve.

*INGREDIENT TIP* Save the juices from the slow cooker after cooking the carnitas so you can drizzle them on top before serving. I also use them when I reheat leftover carnitas in a skillet.

# CARNITAS NACHOS

Pork-rind nachos are absolutely my favorite way to use my slow-cooker Carnitas (page 123). You won't even miss traditional nachos after you taste these. Make the carnitas ahead, and you can whip up a batch of these in no time.

**30-MINUTE**

**SERVES 2**
**PREP** 5 minutes
**COOK** 10 minutes

1 tablespoon olive oil,
plus more for coating

2 cups pork rinds
(I use spicy flavor)

½ cup shredded cheese
(I use Mexican blend)

1 cup Carnitas (page 123)

1 avocado, diced

2 tablespoons sour cream

**Per Batch**
Calories: 1174; Total Fat: 102g;
Carbs: 20g; Net Carbs: 9g;
Fiber: 11g; Protein: 101g

**Per Serving**
Calories: 587; Total Fat: 51g;
Carbs: 10g; Net Carbs: 5g;
Fiber: 6g; Protein: 51g

1. Preheat the oven to 350°F. Coat a 9-by-13-inch baking dish with olive oil.

2. Put the pork rinds in the prepared baking dish, and top with the cheese.

3. Put in the oven and bake until the cheese has melted, about 5 minutes. Transfer to a cooling rack and let rest for 5 minutes.

4. In a medium skillet over high heat, heat the olive oil. Put the carnitas in the skillet, and add some of the reserved pan juices. Cook for a few minutes, until you get a nice crispy crust on the carnitas, and then flip the carnitas to the other side and cook briefly.

5. Divide the heated pork rinds and cheese between two plates.

6. Top the pork rinds and cheese with the reheated carnitas, add the diced avocado and a dollop of sour cream to each, and serve hot.

*INGREDIENT TIP* Keep an eye on the cheese; it won't take very long to melt, and it will continue to melt after you bring the dish out of the oven.

# PEPPERONI LOW-CARB TORTILLA PIZZA

There are so many great ways to make a low-carb pizza, but this version wins for being the quickest and the easiest. My daughter and I sometimes get home late, and this recipe is perfect for such late evenings.

30-MINUTE
ONE PAN

**SERVES 2**
**PREP** 5 minutes
**COOK** 5 minutes

2 tablespoons olive oil

2 large low-carb tortillas
(I use Mission brand)

4 tablespoons low-sugar
tomato sauce (I use Rao's)

1 cup shredded
mozzarella cheese

2 teaspoons dried Italian
seasoning

½ cup pepperoni

**Per Batch**
Calories: 1094; Total Fat: 88g;
Carbs: 34g; Net Carbs: 16g;
Fiber: 18g; Protein: 54g

**Per Serving**
Calories: 547; Total Fat: 44g;
Carbs: 17g; Net Carbs: 8g;
Fiber: 9g; Protein: 27g

1. In a medium skillet over medium-high heat, heat the olive oil. Add the tortilla.

2. Spoon the tomato sauce onto the tortilla, spreading it out. Sprinkle on the cheese, Italian seasoning, and pepperoni. Work quickly so the tortilla doesn't burn.

3. Cook until the tortilla is crispy on the bottom, about 3 minutes. Transfer to a cutting board, and cut into slices. Put the slices on a serving plate and serve hot.

*INGREDIENT TIP*  You can use your favorite low-carb tortilla for this recipe. The olive oil helps make it really crisp so it feels like a pizza.

**VARIATIONS**

Since it's pizza, the possibilities are endless. Here are some of my favorite combinations:

- My favorite version does not use tomato sauce at all, just mozzarella cheese, pepperoni, pepperoncini, and Parmesan cheese.
- Another favorite uses tomato sauce, slices of fresh mozzarella cheese, thin tomato slices, and fresh basil leaves.

# BEEF AND BROCCOLI ROAST

Asian restaurants concern me the most regarding my keto diet because I know many of their sauces have sugar or brown sugar hidden in them. I love making a copycat meal like this roast at home, because I know exactly what's inside. The recipe is not authentic, but it is yummy, and you need only 5 ingredients and a few hours for them in the slow cooker to create tender beef, crisp broccoli, and a salty sauce.

**SERVES 2**
**PREP** 10 minutes
**COOK** 4 hours 30 minutes

1 pound beef chuck roast

Pink Himalayan salt

Freshly ground
black pepper

½ cup beef broth, plus
more if needed

¼ cup soy sauce
(or coconut aminos)

1 teaspoon toasted
sesame oil

1 (16-ounce) bag
frozen broccoli

**Per Batch**
Calories: 1611; Total Fat: 97g;
Carbs: 35g; Net Carbs: 23g;
Fiber: 12g; Protein: 148g

**Per Serving**
Calories: 806; Total Fat: 49g;
Carbs: 18g; Net Carbs: 12g;
Fiber: 6g; Protein: 74g

1. With the crock insert in place, preheat the slow cooker to low.

2. On a cutting board, season the chuck roast with pink Himalayan salt and pepper, and slice the roast thin. Put the sliced beef in the slow cooker.

3. In a small bowl, mix together the beef broth, soy sauce, and sesame oil. Pour over the beef.

4. Cover and cook on low for 4 hours.

5. Add the frozen broccoli, and cook for 30 minutes more. If you need more liquid, add additional beef broth.

6. Serve hot.

*SERVING TIP* I like to spoon this recipe over shirataki rice or cauliflower rice (see Serving Tip, page 120).

# BEEF AND BELL PEPPER "POTATO SKINS"

I love a creative, low-carb take on nachos and other classic game-watching food. I make pork-rind nachos and cauliflower nachos all the time, and then one day I figured I could take pepper slices and make a low-carb version of a potato skin–like dish! The big slices of bell pepper provide the "skin" to hold all the yummy ingredients while also offering a fresh, crisp taste. For additional flavor variations, add Mexican-inspired ingredients like diced onion, diced jalapeño or green chiles, chopped fresh cilantro, freshly squeezed lime juice (for the crema), or hot sauce.

**30-MINUTE**

**SERVES 2**
**PREP** 10 minutes
**COOK** 20 minutes

1 tablespoon ghee

½ pound ground beef

Pink Himalayan salt

Freshly ground
black pepper

3 large bell peppers,
in different colors

½ cup shredded cheese
(I use Mexican blend)

1 avocado

¼ cup sour cream

**Per Batch**
Calories: 1413; Total Fat: 103g;
Carbs: 44g; Net Carbs: 25g;
Fiber: 19g; Protein: 80g

**Per Serving**
Calories: 707; Total Fat: 52g;
Carbs: 22g; Net Carbs: 13g;
Fiber: 10g; Protein: 40g

1. Preheat the oven to 400°F. Line a baking sheet with aluminum foil or a silicone baking mat.

2. In a large skillet over medium-high heat, melt the ghee. When the ghee is hot, add the ground beef and season with pink Himalayan salt and pepper. Stir occasionally with a wooden spoon, breaking up the beef chunks. Continue cooking until the beef
is done, 7 to 10 minutes.

3. Meanwhile, cut the bell peppers to get your "potato skins" ready: Cut off the top of each pepper, slice it in half, and pull out the seeds and ribs. If the pepper is large, you can cut it into quarters; use your best judgment, with the goal of a potato skin–size "boat."

4. Place the bell peppers on the prepared baking sheet.

5. Spoon the ground beef into the peppers, sprinkle the cheese on top of each, and bake for 10 minutes.

6. Meanwhile, in a medium bowl, mix the avocado and sour cream to create an avocado crema. Mix until smooth.

7. When the peppers and beef are done baking, divide them between two plates, top each with the avocado crema, and serve.

*SUBSTITUTION TIP* You could also use ground turkey instead of ground beef.

# SKIRT STEAK WITH CHIMICHURRI SAUCE

This dish has such a bold and savory combination of flavors. The key is marinating the skirt steak as long as you can to get it tender, and then it will melt in your mouth. The sliced steak is then topped with zesty garlic chimichurri sauce before serving, jolting your taste buds into a happy dance.

**SERVES 2**
**PREP** 10 minutes, plus at least all day to marinate
**COOK** 10 minutes

¼ cup soy sauce

½ cup olive oil

Juice of 1 lime

2 tablespoons apple cider vinegar

1 pound skirt steak

Pink Himalayan salt

Freshly ground black pepper

2 tablespoons ghee

¼ cup chimichurri sauce (I use Elvio's)

**Per Batch***
Calories: 1435; Total Fat: 91g; Carbs: 12g; Net Carbs: 8g; Fiber: 4g; Protein: 139g

*This includes 2 tablespoons of soy sauce and olive oil left over in the marinade that is not consumed.

**Per Serving**
Calories: 718; Total Fat: 46g; Carbs: 6g; Net Carbs: 4g; Fiber: 2g; Protein: 70g

1. In a small bowl, mix together the soy sauce, olive oil, lime juice, and apple cider vinegar. Pour into a large zip-top bag, and add the skirt steak. Marinate for as long as possible: at least all day or, ideally, overnight.

2. Dry the steak with a paper towel. Season both sides of the steak with pink Himalayan salt and pepper.

3. In a large skillet over high heat, melt the ghee. Add the steak and sear for about 4 minutes on each side, until well browned. Transfer the steak to a chopping board to rest for at least 5 minutes.

4. Slice the skirt steak against the grain. Divide the slices between two plates, top with the chimichurri sauce, and serve.

*INGREDIENT TIP* You can also make your own chimichurri sauce with a combination of ⅛ cup of cilantro, ⅛ cup of minced red onion, ⅛ cup of chopped parsley, 1 minced garlic clove, 1 tablespoon of olive oil, and 1 tablespoon of apple cider vinegar, and season with pink Himalayan salt and freshly ground black pepper.

# BARBACOA BEEF ROAST

When I see barbacoa, I think of Chipotle restaurant. Their version has 11 or 12 ingredients, but I created one with only 5 ingredients. It is still packed full of flavor, and after 8 hours it will fall apart when you shred it.

**SERVES 2**
**PREP** 10 minutes
**COOK** 8 hours

1 pound beef chuck roast

Pink Himalayan salt

Freshly ground
black pepper

4 chipotle peppers in adobo sauce (I use La Costeña 12-ounce can)

1 (6-ounce) can green jalapeño chiles

2 tablespoons apple cider vinegar

½ cup beef broth

**Per Batch**
Calories: 1446; Total Fat: 91g;
Carbs: 13g; Net Carbs: 3g;
Fiber: 10g; Protein: 131g

**Per Serving**
Calories: 723; Total Fat: 46g;
Carbs: 7g; Net Carbs: 2g;
Fiber: 5g; Protein: 66g

1. With the crock insert in place, preheat the slow cooker to low.

2. Season the beef chuck roast on both sides with pink Himalayan salt
and pepper. Put the roast in the slow cooker.

3. In a food processor (or blender), combine the chipotle peppers and their adobo sauce, jalapeños, and apple cider vinegar, and pulse until smooth. Add the beef broth, and pulse a few more times. Pour the chile mixture over the top of the roast.

4. Cover and cook on low for 8 hours.

5. Transfer the beef to a cutting board, and use two forks to shred the meat.

6. Serve hot.

*INGREDIENT TIP* You can also use beef brisket for this roast.

# STEAK AND EGG BIBIMBAP

*Bibimbap* means "mixed rice" in Korean, and it's one of my favorite Asian dishes. While this recipe is unlike a traditional version, it has the key ingredients: beef, a runny egg, and vegetables. I tend to make this when I have leftovers, because you can really throw in most veggies.

**30-MINUTE**

**SERVES 2**
**PREP** 10 minutes
**COOK** 15 minutes

**FOR THE STEAK**

1 tablespoon ghee or butter

8 ounces skirt steak

Pink Himalayan salt

Freshly ground
black pepper

1 tablespoon soy sauce
(or coconut aminos)

**FOR THE EGG AND
CAULIFLOWER RICE**

2 tablespoons ghee or
butter, divided

2 large eggs

1 large cucumber, peeled
and cut into matchsticks

1 tablespoon soy sauce

1 cup cauliflower rice (see
Serving Tip, page 120)

Pink Himalayan salt

Freshly ground
black pepper

---

**Per Batch**
Calories: 1180; Total Fat: 89g;
Carbs: 16g; Net Carbs: 10g;
Fiber: 7g; Protein: 77g

**Per Serving**
Calories: 590; Total Fat: 45g;
Carbs: 8g; Net Carbs: 5g;
Fiber: 4g; Protein: 39g

**TO MAKE THE STEAK**

1. Over high heat, heat a large skillet.

2. Using a paper towel, pat the steak dry. Season both sides with pink Himalayan salt and pepper.

3. Add the ghee or butter to the skillet. When it melts, put the steak in the skillet.

4. Sear the steak for about 3 minutes on each side for medium-rare.

5. Transfer the steak to a cutting board and let it rest for at least 5 minutes.

6. Slice the skirt steak across the grain and divide it between two bowls.

**TO MAKE THE EGG AND CAULIFLOWER RICE**

1. In a second large skillet over medium-high heat, heat 1 tablespoon of ghee or butter. When the ghee is very hot, crack the eggs into it. When the whites have cooked through, after 2 to 3 minutes, carefully transfer the eggs to a plate.

2. In a small bowl, marinate the cucumber matchsticks in the soy sauce.

3. Clean out the skillet from the eggs, and add the remaining 1 tablespoon of ghee or butter to the pan over medium-high heat. Add the cauliflower rice, season with pink Himalayan salt and pepper, and stir, cooking for 5 minutes. Turn the heat up to high at the end of the cooking to get a nice crisp on the "rice."

4. Divide the rice between two bowls.

5. Top the rice in each bowl with an egg, the steak, and the marinated cucumber matchsticks and serve.

*INGREDIENT TIP* You could also make this recipe with ground turkey or beef instead of steak.

## VARIATIONS

You can add so many vegetables and other ingredients to a bibimbap, so take a look in your fridge and get creative. My favorite add-ins are:

- Kimchi
- Sriracha, drizzled on top
- Bean sprouts
- Carrot matchsticks
- Chopped mushrooms
- Chopped scallions

# MISSISSIPPI POT ROAST

Mississippi Pot Roast is requested on my keto Instagram feed all the time. It is definitely a favorite, because it is so simple and packed with flavor. It also uses one of my favorite ingredients: pepperoncini. Everyone's recipe is a little bit different, but this one reminds me of my mom, because she loves recipes with easy seasoning packets. Here the ranch dressing and gravy packets contribute some excellent flavors.

ONE POT

**SERVES 4**
**PREP** 5 minutes
**COOK** 8 hours

1 pound beef chuck roast

Pink Himalayan salt

Freshly ground
black pepper

1 (1-ounce) packet
dry Au Jus Gravy Mix

1 (1-ounce) packet
dry ranch dressing

8 tablespoons butter
(1 stick)

1 cup whole pepperoncini
(I use Mezzetta)

**Per Batch**
Calories: 2016; Total Fat: 142g;
Carbs: 22g; Net Carbs: 22g;
Fiber: 0g; Protein: 145g

**Per Serving**
Calories: 504; Total Fat: 34g;
Carbs: 6g; Net Carbs: 6g;
Fiber: 0g; Protein: 36g

1. With the crock insert in place, preheat the slow cooker to low.

2. Season both sides of the beef chuck roast with pink Himalayan salt and pepper. Put in the slow cooker.

3. Sprinkle the gravy mix and ranch dressing packets on top of the roast.

4. Place the butter on top of the roast, and sprinkle the pepperoncini around it.

5. Cover and cook on low for 8 hours.

6. Shred the beef using two forks, and serve hot.

*INGREDIENT TIP* You can make this recipe with boneless chicken breasts, and it is delicious.

# TACO CHEESE CUPS

Cheese cups are versatile and very easy to make. Once you master the cheese chips, you will no doubt start making cheese taco shells, cheese bowls, cheese everything! These Mexican-themed taco cups include flavorful beef, fresh avocado, cool sour cream, and of course the crunch of the cheese cup. Delicious and fun to eat!

30-MINUTE

SERVES 2
PREP 10 minutes
COOK 20 minutes

**FOR THE CHEESE CUPS**

2 cups shredded cheese
(I use Mexican blend)

**FOR THE GROUND BEEF**

1 tablespoon ghee

½ pound ground beef

½ (1.25-ounce) package
taco seasoning

¼ cup water

**FOR THE TACO CUPS**

½ avocado, diced

Pink Himalayan salt

Freshly ground
black pepper

2 tablespoons sour cream

**Per Batch**
Calories: 1787; Total Fat: 136g;
Carbs: 23g; Net Carbs: 18g;
Fiber: 5g; Protein: 113g

**Per Serving**
Calories: 894; Total Fat: 68g;
Carbs: 12g; Net Carbs: 9g;
Fiber: 3g; Protein: 57g

**TO MAKE THE CHEESE CUPS**

1. Preheat the oven to 350°F. Line a baking sheet with parchment paper or a silicone baking mat.

2. Place ½-cup mounds of the cheese on the prepared pan. Bake for about 7 minutes, or until the edges are brown and the middle has melted. You want these slightly larger than a typical tortilla chip.

3. Put the pan on a cooling rack for 2 minutes while the cheese chips cool. The chips will be floppy when they first come out of the oven, but they will begin to crisp as they cool.

4. Before they are fully crisp, move the cheese chips to a muffin tin. Form the cheese chips around the shape of the muffin cups to create small bowls. (The chips will fully harden in the muffin tin, which will make them really easy to fill.)

**TO MAKE THE GROUND BEEF**

1. In a medium skillet over medium-high heat, heat the ghee.

2. When the ghee is hot, add the ground beef and sauté for about 8 minutes, until browned.

3. Drain the excess grease. Stir in the taco seasoning and water, and bring to a boil. Turn the heat to medium-low and simmer for 5 minutes.

**TO MAKE THE TACO CUPS**

1.  Using a slotted spoon, spoon the ground beef into the taco cups.

2.  Season the diced avocado with pink Himalayan salt and pepper, and divide it among the taco cups.

3.  Add a dollop of sour cream to each taco cup and serve.

*STORAGE TIP*  The taco cups will keep well for 2 to 3 days in a sealed container in the refrigerator.

**VARIATIONS**

Just like a taco shell, these taco cheese cups can be used to hold any number of flavor combinations:

- Diced tomatoes, onions, and jalapeños can be added to the ground beef.
- Use pepper Jack cheese for an extra kick.

# BACON CHEESEBURGER CASSEROLE

My daughter loves this casserole. It heats up wonderfully as leftovers, so we usually make this once a week during the winter months. This is a hearty, protein-filled dish, so I like to make it on days when I intermittent-fast all day long and just eat dinner.

**SERVES 4**
**PREP** 10 minutes
**COOK** 50 minutes

**FOR THE BACON AND GROUND BEEF**

1 pound bacon

1 tablespoon ghee

1 pound ground beef

Pink Himalayan salt

Freshly ground black pepper

**FOR THE CASSEROLE**

1 tablespoon ghee

½ cup heavy (whipping) cream

4 large eggs, lightly beaten

¾ cup shredded cheese (I use Mexican blend)

Pink Himalayan salt

Freshly ground black pepper

**Per Batch**
Calories: 4706; Total Fat: 363g;
Carbs: 11g; Net Carbs: 11g;
Fiber: 0g; Protein: 330g

**Per Serving**
Calories: 1177; Total Fat: 91g;
Carbs: 3g; Net Carbs: 3g;
Fiber: 0g; Protein: 83g

**TO MAKE THE BACON AND GROUND BEEF**

1. In a large skillet over medium-high heat, cook the bacon on both sides until crispy, about 8 minutes. Transfer the bacon to a paper towel–lined plate to drain and cool for 5 minutes. Transfer to a cutting board and chop the bacon.

2. In a second large skillet over medium-high heat, heat the ghee. Add the ground beef and season with pink Himalayan salt and pepper. Stir occasionally, breaking the beef chunks apart.

3. Once the meat is browned, after about 8 minutes, drain the fat and mix in the chopped bacon.

**TO MAKE THE CASSEROLE**

1. Preheat the oven to 350°F. Coat a 9-by-13-inch baking dish with the ghee.

2. Spoon the meat-and-bacon mixture into the baking dish as a first layer.

3. In a medium bowl, mix together the cream, eggs, and half of the cheese, and season with pink Himalayan salt and pepper. Pour over the meat. Top with the remaining half of the cheese.

→

4.  Bake for 30 minutes, or until the cheese on top is melted and lightly browned.

5.  Let the casserole sit for 5 minutes on a cooling rack before cutting and serving.

*INGREDIENT TIP*  You could also make this recipe with ground turkey instead of ground beef.

## VARIATIONS

I recommend incorporating some of the following variations in the recipe to add some acidity:

- Add diced pickles into the beef mixture. I always do this step because it adds a nice acidity to an otherwise very heavy dish. I use ½ cup of diced pickles.
- Sliced pepperoncini works well, too, if you aren't a fan of pickles.
- Adding a low-sugar tomato sauce like Rao's brand to the cream-and-eggs mixture also provides a nice flavor. I use ¼ cup of tomato sauce.

# FETA-STUFFED BURGERS

Who doesn't love a burger? Especially a burger stuffed with cheese! The combo of the beef and lamb with classic Mediterranean flavors is a winner.

30-MINUTE

**SERVES 2**
**PREP** 10 minutes
**COOK** 10 minutes

2 tablespoons fresh mint leaves, finely chopped

1 scallion, white and green parts, thinly sliced

1 tablespoon Dijon mustard

Pink Himalayan salt

Freshly ground black pepper

12 ounces (6 ounces each) ground beef and ground lamb mixture

2 ounces crumbled feta cheese

1 tablespoon ghee

**Per Batch**
Calories: 1214; Total Fat: 95g; Carbs: 4g; Net Carbs: 3g; Fiber: 1g; Protein: 81g

**Per Serving**
Calories: 607; Total Fat: 48g; Carbs: 2g; Net Carbs: 2g; Fiber: 1g; Protein: 41g

1. In a large bowl, mix to combine the mint leaves with the scallion and mustard. Season with pink Himalayan salt and pepper.

2. Add the ground beef and lamb to the bowl. Mix together thoroughly, and form into 4 patties.

3. Press the feta crumbles into 2 of the patties, and put the other 2 patties on top so the cheese is in the middle. Pinch all the way around the edges of the burgers to seal in the feta cheese.

4. In a medium skillet over medium heat, heat the ghee. Add the burger patties to the hot oil. Cook each side for 4 to 5 minutes, until done to your preference, and serve.

*SUBSTITUTION TIP* You could use just ground beef or just ground lamb for this recipe if you prefer.

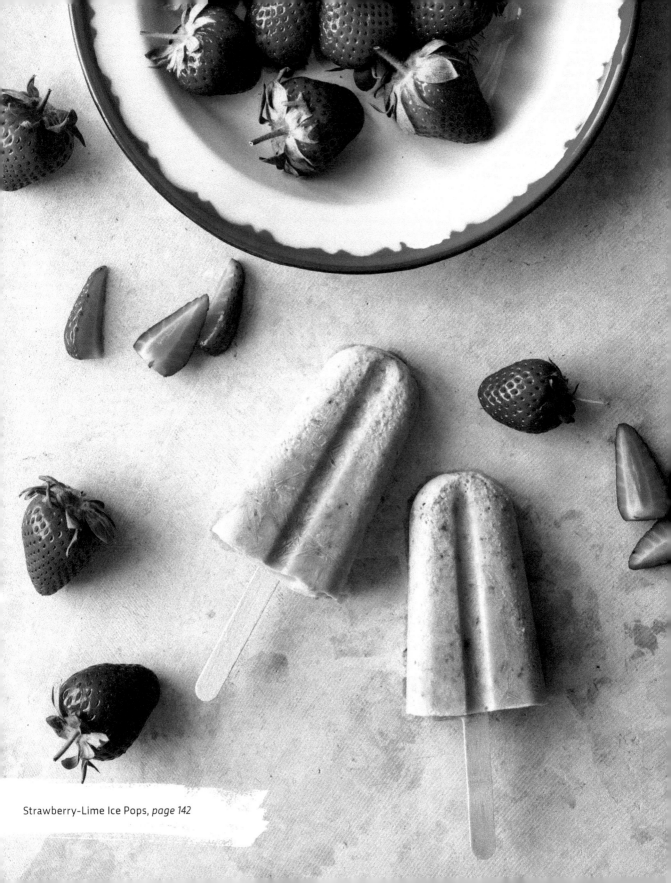

Strawberry-Lime Ice Pops, *page 142*

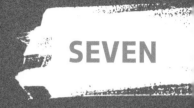

# SEVEN

# DESSERTS & SWEET TREATS

Desserts can be fun on a keto diet! I try to keep my dessert recipes as simple as possible so that if I am craving something sweet I can prepare a recipe quickly with ingredients I already have in the house. I make dessert an occasional treat, maybe once a week, because I find that the less I eat sweet foods, the less I crave them. Keep things simple with these 5-ingredient keto desserts.

# BLUEBERRY-BLACKBERRY ICE POPS

Blueberries are my favorite fruit, and blackberries are a close second. So I created a creamy, refreshing ice pop using both. The color of these ice pops is gorgeous!

NO COOK
VEGETARIAN

**SERVES 2**
**PREP** 5 minutes, plus at least 2 hours to freeze

½ (13.5-ounce) can coconut cream, ¾ cup unsweetened full-fat coconut milk, or ¾ cup heavy (whipping) cream

2 teaspoons Swerve natural sweetener or 2 drops liquid stevia

½ teaspoon vanilla extract

¼ cup mixed blueberries and blackberries (fresh or frozen)

**Per Batch**
Calories: 661; Total Fat: 68g; Carbs: 17g; Net Carbs: 7g; Fiber: 2g; Protein: 4g

**Per Serving**
Calories: 165; Total Fat: 17g; Carbs: 4g; Net Carbs: 2g; Fiber: 1g; Protein: 1g

1. In a food processor (or blender), mix together the coconut cream, sweetener, and vanilla.

2. Add the mixed berries, and pulse just a few times so the blueberries retain their texture.

3. Pour into ice pop molds and freeze for at least 2 hours before serving.

*INGREDIENT TIP* If you don't have both blueberries and blackberries, you can make this recipe with just one or the other.

# STRAWBERRY-LIME ICE POPS

The fresh, delicious flavors of this ice pop remind me of a Mexican *paleta*. I love the addition of lime juice so that you have sweet, creamy, and sour flavors all in one delicious ice pop.

NO COOK
VEGETARIAN

**SERVES 4**
**PREP** 5 minutes,
plus at least 2 hours
to freeze

½ (13.5-ounce) can
coconut cream, ¾ cup
unsweetened full-fat
coconut milk, or ¾ cup
heavy (whipping) cream

2 teaspoons Swerve
natural sweetener or
2 drops liquid stevia

1 tablespoon freshly
squeezed lime juice

¼ cup hulled and sliced
strawberries (fresh
or frozen)

**Per Batch**
Calories: 663; Total Fat: 68g;
Carbs: 20g; Net Carbs: 10g;
Fiber: 2g; Protein: 4g

**Per Serving**
Calories: 166; Total Fat: 17g;
Carbs: 5g; Net Carbs: 3g;
Fiber: 1g; Protein: 1g

1. In a food processor (or blender), mix together the coconut cream, sweetener, and lime juice.

2. Add the strawberries, and pulse just a few times so the strawberries retain their texture.

3. Pour into ice pop molds, and freeze for at least 2 hours before serving.

*INGREDIENT TIP* You can also replace the strawberries with blackberries.

# COFFEE ICE POPS

Coffee is a staple for so many people on a keto diet. Why not freeze it into a convenient ice pop form? The mix of coffee and cream is extra fun with the addition of sugar-free chocolate chips.

NO COOK
VEGETARIAN

**SERVES 4**
**PREP** 5 minutes,
plus 2 hours to freeze

2 cups brewed coffee, cold

¾ cup coconut cream,
¾ cup unsweetened full-fat
coconut milk, or ¾ cup
heavy (whipping) cream

2 teaspoons Swerve
natural sweetener or
2 drops liquid stevia

2 tablespoons sugar-free
chocolate chips (I use Lily's)

**Per Batch**
Calories: 419; Total Fat: 41g;
Carbs: 29g; Net Carbs: 7g;
Fiber: 8g; Protein: 4g

**Per Serving**
Calories: 105; Total Fat: 10g;
Carbs: 7g; Net Carbs: 2g;
Fiber: 2g; Protein: 1g

1. In a food processor (or blender), mix together the coffee, coconut cream, and sweetener until thoroughly blended.

2. Pour into ice pop molds, and drop a few chocolate chips into each mold.

3. Freeze for at least 2 hours before serving.

*INGREDIENT TIP* You can adjust the sweetness to your personal taste.

**VARIATIONS**
You can add in your favorite sugar-free flavorings, to customize the ice pops just as you would your coffee:

- Cinnamon
- Vanilla
- Chocolate protein powder

# FUDGE ICE POPS

Ice pops are one of my favorite desserts because it's simple to make a batch, and then I have something sweet ready for that occasional craving. Ice pops are also a fun way to get creative with different flavors. I recommend investing in good-quality ice pop molds.

**NO COOK**
**VEGETARIAN**

**SERVES 4**
**PREP** 5 minutes,
plus 2 hours to freeze

½ (13.5-ounce) can coconut cream, ¾ cup unsweetened full-fat coconut milk, or ¾ cup heavy (whipping) cream

2 teaspoons Swerve natural sweetener or 2 drops liquid stevia

2 tablespoons unsweetened cocoa powder

2 tablespoons sugar-free chocolate chips (I use Lily's)

**Per Batch**
Calories: 771; Total Fat: 79g;
Carbs: 37g; Net Carbs: 13g;
Fiber: 10g; Protein: 8g

**Per Serving**
Calories: 193; Total Fat: 20g;
Carbs: 9g; Net Carbs: 3g;
Fiber: 3g; Protein: 2g

1. In a food processor (or blender), mix together the coconut cream, sweetener, and unsweetened cocoa powder.

2. Pour into ice pop molds, and drop chocolate chips into each mold.

3. Freeze for at least 2 hours before serving.

*INGREDIENT TIP* You can adjust the sweetness to your personal taste.

**VARIATIONS**
Have fun playing with the mix-ins:
- You can add collagen powder to the mix for added health benefits.
- Choose the heavy (whipping) cream and add cream cheese. Fold in the chocolate chips at the end of the recipe.

# ROOT BEER FLOAT

I remember the day I realized I could easily make a keto-friendly root beer float. So exciting! This version is keto-friendly, and you won't miss the sugar, at all.

30-MINUTE
ONE PAN
NO COOK
VEGETARIAN

**SERVES 2**

**PREP** 5 minutes

1 (12-ounce) can diet root beer (I like Zevia's)

4 tablespoons heavy (whipping) cream

1 teaspoon vanilla extract

6 ice cubes

**Per Batch**
Calories: 111; Total Fat: 11g;
Carbs: 5g; Net Carbs: 1g;
Fiber: 0g; Protein: 1g

**Per Serving**
Calories: 56; Total Fat: 6g;
Carbs: 3g; Net Carbs: 1g;
Fiber: 0g; Protein: 1g

1. In a food processor (or blender), combine the root beer, cream, vanilla, and ice.

2. Blend well, pour into two tall glasses, and serve.

3. For me, no root beer float is complete without a bendy straw.

*INGREDIENT TIP* If you are looking for a boozy root beer float, you can add vanilla vodka or rum to this mix.

# ORANGE CREAM FLOAT

Orange is not a flavor you get to experience very often on the keto diet. That's why I was so excited when I discovered Zevia's Orange Soda made with stevia.

**30-MINUTE**
**ONE PAN**
**NO COOK**
**VEGETARIAN**

**SERVES 2**
**PREP** 5 minutes

1 can diet orange soda
(I like Zevia's)

4 tablespoons heavy
(whipping) cream

1 teaspoon vanilla extract

6 ice cubes

**Per Batch**
Calories: 111; Total Fat: 11g;
Carbs: 5g; Net Carbs: 1g;
Fiber: 0g; Protein: 1g

**Per Serving**
Calories: 56; Total Fat: 6g;
Carbs: 3g; Net Carbs: 1g;
Fiber: 0g; Protein: 1g

1. In a food processor (or blender), combine the orange soda, cream, vanilla, and ice.

2. Blend well, pour into two tall glasses, and serve.

*INGREDIENT TIP* If you're after a boozy orange cream treat, add vanilla vodka to this mix.

# STRAWBERRY SHAKE

Just by looking at the recipe titles in this chapter, you have probably noticed that I love cheese-cake. So why not a strawberry cheesecake–inspired shake? No baking or waiting for anything to set. Just whip it up—ready in minutes!

**30-MINUTE**
**ONE PAN**
**NO COOK**
**VEGETARIAN**

**SERVES 2**
**PREP** 10 minutes

¾ cup heavy
(whipping) cream

2 ounces cream cheese,
at room temperature

1 tablespoon Swerve
natural sweetener

¼ teaspoon vanilla extract

6 strawberries, sliced

6 ice cubes

**Per Batch**
Calories: 813; Total Fat: 83g;
Carbs: 25g; Net Carbs: 11g;
Fiber: 1g; Protein: 7g

**Per Serving**
Calories: 407; Total Fat: 42g;
Carbs: 13g; Net Carbs: 6g;
Fiber: 1g; Protein: 4g

1. In a food processor (or blender), combine the heavy cream, cream cheese, sweetener, and vanilla. Mix on high to fully combine.

2. Add the strawberries and ice, and blend until smooth.

3. Pour into two tall glasses and serve.

*INGREDIENT TIP* A little swirl of whipped cream is always a nice topping to any milkshake.

# "FROSTY" CHOCOLATE SHAKE

I cringe when I think about some of the things I used to eat prior to keto, but one treat I loved to indulge in was a Frosty at Wendy's. Luckily for me, this copycat keto recipe gets really close to the real thing. For the coconut milk, I use part of a 13.5-ounce can of Trader Joe's organic coconut milk, which I stir up after opening. I suggest chilling a medium metal mixing bowl and the hand-mixer beaters in the freezer while you prepare to make this recipe.

ONE PAN
NO COOK
VEGETARIAN

**SERVES 2**
**PREP** 10 minutes,
plus 1 hour to chill

¾ cup heavy
(whipping) cream

4 ounces coconut milk

1 tablespoon Swerve
natural sweetener

¼ teaspoon vanilla extract

2 tablespoons unsweetened
cocoa powder

**Per Batch**
Calories: 887; Total Fat: 93g;
Carbs: 29g; Net Carbs: 13g;
Fiber: 4g; Protein: 8g

**Per Serving**
Calories: 444; Total Fat: 47g;
Carbs: 15g; Net Carbs: 7g;
Fiber: 2g; Protein: 4g

1. Pour the cream into a medium cold metal bowl, and with your hand mixer and cold beaters, beat the cream just until it forms peaks.

2. Slowly pour in the coconut milk, and gently stir it into the cream. Add the sweetener, vanilla, and cocoa powder, and beat until fully combined.

3. Pour into two tall glasses, and chill in the freezer for 1 hour before serving. I usually stir the shakes twice during this time.

*INGREDIENT TIP* Almond milk will work if you don't have coconut milk.

# STRAWBERRY CHEESECAKE MOUSSE

I love this super-easy dessert that any cheesecake-loving person will devour! It takes only 10 minutes to make and can easily be customized with different fruits.

ONE PAN
NO COOK
VEGETARIAN

**SERVES 2**
**PREP** 10 minutes, plus
1 hour to chill

4 ounces cream cheese, at room temperature

1 tablespoon heavy (whipping) cream

1 teaspoon Swerve natural sweetener or 1 drop liquid stevia

1 teaspoon vanilla extract

4 strawberries, sliced (fresh or frozen)

**Per Batch**
Calories: 441; Total Fat: 42g;
Carbs: 21g; Net Carbs: 8g;
Fiber: 1g; Protein: 7g

**Per Serving**
Calories: 221; Total Fat: 21g;
Carbs: 11g; Net Carbs: 4g;
Fiber: 1g; Protein: 4g

1. Break up the cream cheese block into smaller pieces and distribute evenly in a food processor (or blender). Add the cream, sweetener, and vanilla.

2. Mix together on high. I usually stop and stir twice and scrape down the sides of the bowl with a small rubber scraper to make sure everything is mixed well.

3. Add the strawberries to the food processor, and mix until combined.

4. Divide the strawberry cheesecake mixture between two small dishes, and chill for 1 hour before serving.

*INGREDIENT TIP* The heavy whipping cream helps thin out the cream cheese a bit. If it still seems thick when you are mixing, mix in a little more cream.

**VARIATIONS**
- I often use blackberries instead of strawberries, about ¼ cup.
- At winter holidays, instead of strawberries, I love to add 3 ounces of pumpkin purée to this mixture along with 1 teaspoon of pumpkin pie spice.

# LEMONADE FAT BOMB

Fat bombs are a keto thing. When I first started keto, I kept seeing these different fat bomb options, so I had to develop a couple of my own. This lemonade version is a favorite of my daughter's, who loves anything lemon. Let the ingredients sit on the counter for about 2 hours to come to room temperature before you start preparing this recipe. An important step to keep in mind for any fat bomb recipe.

NO COOK
VEGETARIAN

**SERVES 2**
**PREP** 10 minutes, plus 2 hours to freeze

½ lemon

4 ounces cream cheese, at room temperature

2 ounces butter, at room temperature

2 teaspoons Swerve natural sweetener or 2 drops liquid stevia

Pinch pink Himalayan salt

**Per Batch**
Calories: 807; Total Fat: 85g; Carbs: 15g; Net Carbs: 7g; Fiber: 1g; Protein: 8g

**Per Serving**
Calories: 404; Total Fat: 43g; Carbs: 8g; Net Carbs: 4g; Fiber: 1g; Protein: 4g

1. Zest the lemon half with a very fine grater into a small bowl. Squeeze the juice from the lemon half into the bowl with the zest.

2. In a medium bowl, combine the cream cheese and butter. Add the sweetener, lemon zest and juice, and pink Himalayan salt. Using a hand mixer, beat until fully combined.

3. Spoon the mixture into the fat bomb molds. (I use small silicone cupcake molds. If you don't have molds, you can use cupcake paper liners that fit into the cups of a muffin tin.)

4. Freeze for at least 2 hours, unmold, and eat! Keep extras in your freezer in a zip-top bag so you and your loved ones can have them anytime you are craving a sweet treat. They will keep in the freezer for up to 3 months.

*COOKING TIP* You can use an ice cube tray as a super-easy mold for making fat bombs.

# BERRY CHEESECAKE FAT BOMB

These fat bombs give you all the flavor of cheesecake in a small bite. I love the berries in this recipe. I use a combination of strawberries and blackberries, mash them together, and then fold them into the mixture. All ingredients should be room temperature for a fat bomb recipe—an important step for making successful fat bombs.

NO COOK
VEGETARIAN

**SERVES 2**
**PREP** 10 minutes, plus at least 2 hours to freeze

4 ounces cream cheese, at room temperature

4 tablespoons (½ stick) butter, at room temperature

2 teaspoons Swerve natural sweetener or 2 drops liquid stevia

1 teaspoon vanilla extract

¼ cup berries, fresh or frozen

**Per Batch**
Calories: 827; Total Fat: 85g;
Carbs: 17g; Net Carbs: 7g;
Fiber: 2g; Protein: 8g

**Per Serving**
Calories: 414; Total Fat: 43g;
Carbs: 9g; Net Carbs: 4g;
Fiber: 1g; Protein: 4g

1. In a medium bowl, use a hand mixer to beat the cream cheese, butter, sweetener, and vanilla.

2. In a small bowl, mash the berries thoroughly. Fold the berries into the cream-cheese mixture using a rubber scraper. (If you put slices of berries in the cream-cheese mixture without mashing them, they will freeze and have an off-putting texture.)

3. Spoon the cream-cheese mixture into fat bomb molds. (I use small silicone cupcake molds, which I put in the cups of a muffin tin. You can just use cupcake papers if you don't have molds.)

4. Freeze for at least 2 hours, unmold them, and eat! Leftover fat bombs can be stored in the freezer in a zip-top bag for up to 3 months. It's nice to have some in your freezer for when you are craving a sweet treat.

*COOKING TIP* You can use an ice cube tray as an easy fat bomb mold.

# PEANUT BUTTER FAT BOMB

My daughter is a peanut-butter nut, so these fat bombs are an easy way to make her very happy. You can mix these up before you make dinner, and they will be ready in time for dessert: quick and easy. All ingredients should be at room temperature; this is important for any fat bomb recipe.

**VEGETARIAN**

**SERVES 2**

**PREP** 10 minutes, plus 30 minutes to freeze

1 tablespoon butter, at room temperature

1 tablespoon coconut oil

2 tablespoons all-natural peanut butter or almond butter

2 teaspoons Swerve natural sweetener or 2 drops liquid stevia

**Per Batch**
Calories: 391; Total Fat: 39g; Carbs: 15g; Net Carbs: 5g; Fiber: 2g; Protein: 6g

**Per Serving**
Calories: 196; Total Fat: 20g; Carbs: 8g; Net Carbs: 3g; Fiber: 1g; Protein: 3g

1. In a microwave-safe medium bowl, melt the butter, coconut oil, and peanut butter in the microwave on 50 percent power. Mix in the sweetener.

2. Pour the mixture into fat bomb molds. (I use small silicone cupcake molds.)

3. Freeze for 30 minutes, unmold them, and eat! Keep some extras in your freezer so you can eat them anytime you are craving a sweet treat.

*COOKING TIP*  You can use an ice cube tray as a fat bomb mold. When the fat bombs have frozen, take them out of the ice tray, put in a zip-top bag, and store in the freezer for up to 3 months.

# CRUSTLESS CHEESECAKE BITES

Cheesecake is my favorite dessert. Fortunately, it is easy to make keto-friendly cheesecake! These make perfect bite-size desserts for family dinners or for a take-along to a dinner party.

ONE PAN
VEGETARIAN

**SERVES 4**
**PREP** 10 minutes, plus 3 hours to chill
**COOK** 30 minutes

4 ounces cream cheese, at room temperature

¼ cup sour cream

2 large eggs

⅓ cup Swerve natural sweetener

¼ teaspoon vanilla extract

**Per Batch**
Calories: 677; Total Fat: 60g; Carbs: 71g; Net Carbs: 7g; Fiber: 0g; Protein: 20g

**Per Serving**
Calories: 169; Total Fat: 15g; Carbs: 18g; Net Carbs: 2g; Fiber: 0g; Protein: 5g

1. Preheat the oven to 350°F.

2. In a medium mixing bowl, use a hand mixer to beat the cream cheese, sour cream, eggs, sweetener, and vanilla until well mixed.

3. Place silicone liners (or cupcake paper liners) in the cups of a muffin tin.

4. Pour the cheesecake batter into the liners, and bake for 30 minutes.

5. Refrigerate until completely cooled before serving, about 3 hours. Store extra cheesecake bites in a zip-top bag in the freezer for up to 3 months.

*INGREDIENT TIP* I find it much easier to mix the cream cheese when you allow it to come to room temperature.

**VARIATIONS**
- Add lemon zest for a delicious burst of flavor.
- For a keto-friendly version of key lime cheesecake, add ½ teaspoon of sugar-free lime Jello mix and ½ teaspoon of freshly squeezed lime juice to this recipe.

# PUMPKIN CRUSTLESS CHEESECAKE BITES

These bites have classic cheesecake flavor with a pumpkin twist. Perfect for fall, when you're craving all things pumpkin. But equally delicious any time of the year.

VEGETARIAN

**SERVES 4**
**PREP** 10 minutes, plus 3 hours to chill
**COOK** 30 minutes

4 ounces pumpkin purée

4 ounces cream cheese, at room temperature

2 large eggs

⅓ cup Swerve natural sweetener

2 teaspoons pumpkin pie spice

**Per Batch**
Calories: 622; Total Fat: 49g; Carbs: 82g; Net Carbs: 15g; Fiber: 3g; Protein: 21g

**Per Serving**
Calories: 156; Total Fat: 12g; Carbs: 21g; Net Carbs: 4g; Fiber: 1g; Protein: 5g

1. Preheat the oven to 350°F.

2. In a medium mixing bowl, use a hand mixer to mix the pumpkin purée, cream cheese, eggs, sweetener, and pumpkin pie spice until thoroughly combined.

3. Place silicone liners (or cupcake paper liners) into the cups of a muffin tin.

4. Pour the batter into the liners, and bake for 30 minutes.

5. Refrigerate until completely cooled before serving, about 3 hours. Put leftover cheesecake bites in a zip-top plastic bag and store in the freezer for up to 3 months.

*INGREDIENT TIP* You'll want to use pure pumpkin for this recipe, not pumpkin pie mix, which has added sugar.

# BERRY-PECAN MASCARPONE BOWL

A lot of people enjoy this dish for breakfast, but with cottage cheese. I tried it one night with mascarpone with a touch of sweetener and loved it; it felt like a real dessert. Then I added in a small handful of keto-friendly chocolate chips, and I was in dessert heaven.

30-MINUTE
ONE PAN
NO COOK
VEGETARIAN

**SERVES 2**
**PREP** 5 minutes

1 cup chopped pecans

1 teaspoon Swerve natural sweetener or 1 drop liquid stevia

¼ cup mascarpone

30 Lily's dark-chocolate chips

6 strawberries, sliced

**Per Batch**
Calories: 923; Total Fat: 93g; Carbs: 30g; Net Carbs: 11g; Fiber: 14g; Protein: 12g

**Per Serving**
Calories: 462; Total Fat: 47g; Carbs: 15g; Net Carbs: 6g; Fiber: 7g; Protein: 6g

1. Divide the pecans between two dessert bowls.

2. In a small bowl, mix the sweetener into the mascarpone cheese. Top the nuts with a dollop of the sweetened mascarpone.

3. Sprinkle in the chocolate chips, top each dish with the strawberries, and serve.

*SUBSTITUTION TIP* You could also use ricotta cheese instead of mascarpone.

# PEANUT BUTTER COOKIES

If you like peanut butter, you will love these cookies. They are very simple, using just three ingredients. Maybe it is my keto taste buds, but to me these cookies taste just like the full-sugar version!

30-MINUTE
VEGETARIAN

Makes 15 cookies
**PREP** 5 minutes
**COOK** 10 minutes, plus
10 minutes to cool

1 cup natural crunchy
peanut butter

½ cup Swerve
natural sweetener

1 egg

**Per Batch**
Calories: 1466; Total Fat: 118g;
Carbs: 153g; Net Carbs: 43g;
Fiber: 14g; Protein: 56g

**Per Cookie**
Calories: 98; Total Fat: 8g;
Carbs: 10g; Net Carbs: 3g;
Fiber: 1g; Protein: 4g

1. Preheat the oven to 350°F. Line a baking sheet with a silicone baking mat or parchment paper.

2. In a medium bowl, use a hand mixer to mix together the peanut butter, sweetener, and egg.

3. Roll up the batter into small balls about 1 inch in diameter.

4. Spread out the cookie-dough balls on the prepared pan. Press each dough ball down with the tines of a fork, then repeat to make a crisscross pattern.

5. Bake for about 12 minutes, or until golden.

6. Let the cookies cool for 10 minutes on the lined pan before serving. If you try to move them too soon, they will crumble.

7. Store leftover cookies covered in the refrigerator for up to 5 days.

*INGREDIENT TIP* You can use creamy peanut butter, but I think the texture of the nuts makes for a better cookie.

# CHOCOLATE MOUSSE

This dessert is rich, chocolatey, and super indulgent. It is packed with fats and bursting with creamy, chocolatey flavor.

NO COOK
VEGETARIAN

**SERVES 2**
**PREP** 10 minutes,
plus 1 hour to chill

1½ tablespoons heavy (whipping) cream

4 tablespoons butter, at room temperature

1 tablespoon unsweetened cocoa powder

4 tablespoons cream cheese, at room temperature

1 tablespoon Swerve natural sweetener

**Per Batch**
Calories: 920; Total Fat: 99g;
Carbs: 20g; Net Carbs: 7g;
Fiber: 1g; Protein: 7g

**Per Serving**
Calories: 460; Total Fat: 50g;
Carbs: 10g; Net Carbs: 4g;
Fiber: 1g; Protein: 4g

1. In a medium chilled bowl, use a whisk or fork to whip the cream. Refrigerate to keep cold.

2. In a separate medium bowl, use a hand mixer to beat the butter, cocoa powder, cream cheese, and sweetener until thoroughly combined.

3. Take the whipped cream out of the refrigerator. Gently fold the whipped cream into the chocolate mixture with a rubber scraper.

4. Divide the pudding between two dessert bowls.

5. Cover and chill for 1 hour before serving.

*COOKING TIP* For making the whipping cream, I like to leave a clean medium metal bowl in the freezer for a couple of hours before I use it. If using beaters, you can also put those in the freezer to chill for a few minutes before whipping the cream.

**VARIATIONS**
Chocolate pairs well with a variety of flavors and textures:
- Fresh raspberries are delicious on top of this mousse.
- For extra-high-quality fat, I like to add ¼ of an avocado to this mix. The avocado adds a smooth creaminess.

# MINT–CHOCOLATE CHIP ICE CREAM

There are many low-carbohydrate ice creams on the market these days, but nothing beats making your own. You don't have to have a fancy ice cream maker at home to make this ice cream.

ONE PAN
VEGETARIAN

**SERVES 2**
**PREP** 10 minutes, plus at least 4 hours to freeze
**COOK** 30 minutes

½ tablespoon butter

1 tablespoon Swerve natural sweetener

10 tablespoons heavy (whipping) cream, divided

¼ teaspoon peppermint extract

2 tablespoons sugar-free chocolate chips (I use Lily's)

**Per Batch**
Calories: 650; Total Fat: 66g; Carbs: 34g; Net Carbs: 8g; Fiber: 8g; Protein: 5g

**Per Serving**
Calories: 325; Total Fat: 33g; Carbs: 17g; Net Carbs: 4g; Fiber: 4g; Protein: 3g

1. Put a medium metal bowl and your hand-mixer beaters in the freezer to chill.

2. In a small, heavy saucepan over medium heat, melt the butter. Whisk in the sweetener and 5 tablespoons of cream.

3. Turn the heat up to medium-high and bring the mixture to a boil, stirring constantly. Turn the heat down to low and simmer, stirring occasionally, for about 30 minutes. You want the mixture to be thick, so it sticks to the back of a spoon.

4. Stir in the peppermint extract.

5. Pour the thickened mixture into a medium bowl and refrigerate to cool.

6. Remove the metal bowl and the mixer beaters from the freezer. Pour the remaining 5 tablespoons of cream into the bowl. With the electric beater, whip the cream until it is thick and fluffy and forms peaks. Don't overbeat, or the cream will turn to butter. Take the cream mixture out of the refrigerator.

7. Using a rubber scraper, gently fold the whipped cream into the cooled mixture.

8. Transfer the mixture to a small metal container that can go in the freezer (I use a mini loaf pan since I only make enough for two).

9. Mix in the chocolate chips, and cover the container with foil or plastic wrap.

10. Freeze the ice cream for 4 to 5 hours before serving, stirring it twice during that time.

*SUBSTITUTION TIP* If you don't care for peppermint extract, you can replace it with vanilla extract to make chocolate-chip ice cream.

# CHOCOLATE-AVOCADO PUDDING

I came to this recipe after some trial and error with chocolate-and-avocado creations. I was about to give up on the combination because they just never came out right. Until I discovered this pudding recipe—simple and effective.

ONE PAN
NO COOK
VEGETARIAN

**SERVES 2**
**PREP** 5 minutes, plus
30 minutes to chill

1 ripe medium avocado,
cut into chunks

2 ounces cream cheese,
at room temperature

1 tablespoon Swerve
natural sweetener

4 tablespoons unsweetened
cocoa powder

¼ teaspoon vanilla extract

Pinch pink Himalayan salt

**Per Batch**
Calories: 562; Total Fat: 54g;
Carbs: 54g; Net Carbs: 24g;
Fiber: 19g; Protein: 16g

**Per Serving**
Calories: 281; Total Fat: 27g;
Carbs: 27g; Net Carbs: 12g;
Fiber: 10g; Protein: 8g

1. In a food processor (or blender), combine the avocado with the cream cheese, sweetener, cocoa powder, vanilla, and pink Himalayan salt. Blend until completely smooth.

2. Pour into two small dessert bowls, and chill for 30 minutes before serving.

*INGREDIENT TIP* If you have an extra-large avocado, only use half. You don't want the avocado flavor to be too overwhelming.

# DARK-CHOCOLATE STRAWBERRY BARK

One night I had an urge for some dark chocolate. My daughter uses the keto-friendly dark-chocolate bars melted with heavy whipping cream when she makes chocolate-covered strawberries, so I decided to try something with a little crunch.

VEGETARIAN

**SERVES 2**
**PREP** 10 minutes,
plus 2 hours to chill
**COOK** 1 minute

½ (2.8-ounce) keto-friendly chocolate bar (I use Lily's)
1 tablespoon heavy (whipping) cream
2 tablespoons salted almonds
1 fresh strawberry, sliced

**Per Batch**
Calories: 221; Total Fat: 20g;
Carbs: 17g; Net Carbs: 8g;
Fiber: 9g; Protein: 5g

**Per Serving**
Calories: 111; Total Fat: 10g;
Carbs: 9g; Net Carbs: 4g;
Fiber: 5g; Protein: 3g

1. Line a baking sheet with parchment paper.

2. Break up the chocolate bar half into small pieces, and put them in a microwave-safe bowl with the cream.

3. Heat in the microwave for 45 seconds at 50 percent power. Stir the chocolate, and cook for 20 seconds more at 50 percent power. Stir again, making sure the mixture is fully melted and combined. If not, microwave for another 20 seconds.

4. Pour the chocolate mixture onto the parchment paper and spread it in a thin, uniform layer.

5. Sprinkle on the almonds, then add the strawberry slices.

6. Refrigerate until hardened, about 2 hours.

7. Once the bark is nice and hard, break it up into smaller pieces to nibble on. Yum!

8. The bark will keep for up to 4 days in a sealed container in the refrigerator.

*INGREDIENT TIP* You could substitute macadamia nuts for the almonds in this dessert. It would be a delicious option.

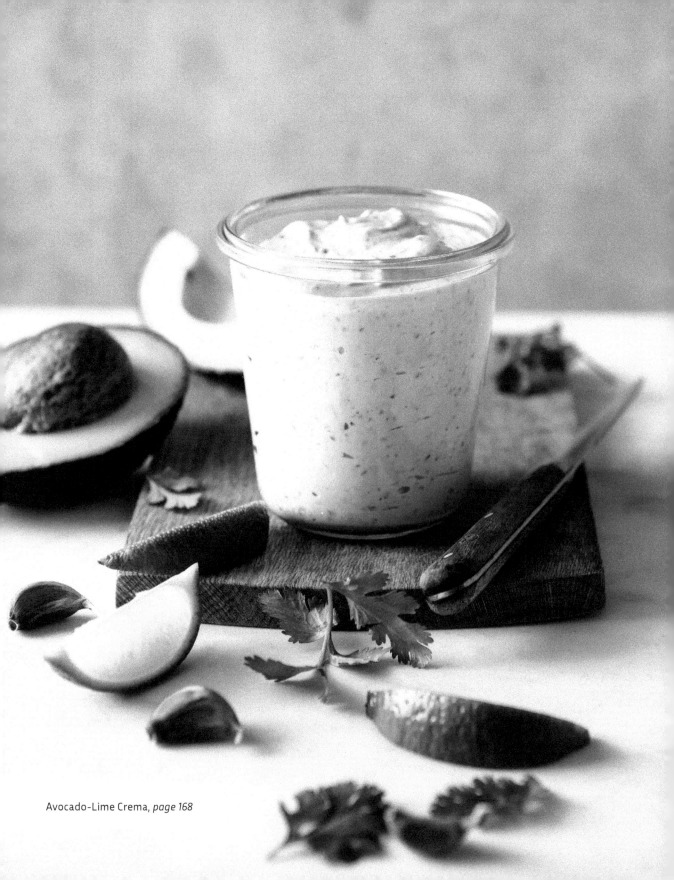

Avocado-Lime Crema, *page 168*

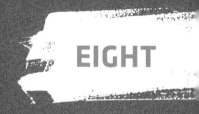

# EIGHT

# SAUCES & DRESSINGS

There are a lot of great low-carb options when it comes to sauces and dressings, but sometimes if you have the ingredients at home, it can be great to make your own. The sauces in this chapter are some of my favorites and generally use ingredients you may already have in your fridge or pantry. The biggest benefit of making your own sauces and dressings, of course, is that you completely control what goes into them, and so can feel confident about their carb count.

# DIJON VINAIGRETTE

I love this light, tangy dressing on salads. It is especially good with salads that have tomatoes, berries, or other sweet elements that the Dijon mustard plays really well with.

**30-MINUTE**

**ONE PAN**

**NO COOK**

**VEGETARIAN**

**SERVES 4**

**PREP** 5 minutes

2 tablespoons
Dijon mustard

Juice of ½ lemon

1 garlic clove, finely minced

1½ tablespoons red
wine vinegar

Pink Himalayan salt

Freshly ground
black pepper

3 tablespoons olive oil

**Per Batch**
Calories: 396; Total Fat: 42g;
Carbs: 5g; Net Carbs: 4g;
Fiber: 2g; Protein: 2g

**Per Serving**
Calories: 99; Total Fat: 11g;
Carbs: 1g; Net Carbs: 1g;
Fiber: 1g; Protein: 1g

1. In a small bowl, whisk the mustard, lemon juice, garlic, and red wine vinegar until well combined. Season with pink Himalayan salt and pepper, and whisk again.

2. Slowly add the olive oil, a little bit at a time, whisking constantly.

3. Keep in a sealed glass container in the refrigerator for up to 1 week.

*SUBSTITUTION TIP* Feel free to replace the red wine vinegar with apple cider vinegar.

# GREEN GODDESS DRESSING

This simple dressing can be made in a flash and tastes absolutely divine when poured over salads and meaty main dishes. Try it over medallions of boneless beef top sirloin that have been grilled and cut into thick slices.

30-MINUTE
ONE POT
NO COOK
VEGETARIAN

**SERVES 4**
**PREP** 5 minutes

2 tablespoon buttermilk

¼ cup Greek yogurt

1 teaspoon apple
cider vinegar

1 garlic clove, minced

1 tablespoon olive oil

1 tablespoon fresh
parsley leaves

**Per Batch**
Calories: 249; Total Fat: 25g;
Carbs: 4g; Net Carbs: 4g;
Fiber: 0g; Protein: 3g

**Per Serving**
Calories: 62; Total Fat: 6g;
Carbs: 1g; Net Carbs: 1g;
Fiber: 0g; Protein: 1g

1. In a food processor (or blender), combine the buttermilk, yogurt, apple cider vinegar, garlic, olive oil, and parsley. Blend until fully combined.

2. Pour into a sealed glass container and chill in the refrigerator for at least 30 minutes before serving. This dressing will keep in the fridge for up to 1 week.

*SUBSTITUTION TIP* This dressing is also delicious if you use sour cream in place of the Greek yogurt, or if you mix some fresh chopped chives in with the parsley.

# CAESAR DRESSING

Caesar is a perfect salad dressing for the keto diet. It is filled with healthy fats and delicious savory ingredients. This dressing can bring a bit of a gourmet feel to even the most basic salad.

30-MINUTE
ONE PAN
NO COOK

**SERVES 4**
**PREP** 5 minutes

½ cup mayonnaise

1 tablespoon Dijon mustard

Juice of ½ lemon

½ teaspoon
Worcestershire sauce

Pinch pink Himalayan salt

Pinch freshly ground
black pepper

¼ cup grated
Parmesan cheese

**Per Batch**
Calories: 889; Total Fat: 93g;
Carbs: 8g; Net Carbs: 7g;
Fiber: 1g; Protein: 9g

**Per Serving**
Calories: 222; Total Fat: 23g;
Carbs: 2g; Net Carbs: 2g;
Fiber: 0g; Protein: 2g

1. In a medium bowl, whisk together the mayonnaise, mustard, lemon juice, Worcestershire sauce, pink Himalayan salt,
and pepper until fully combined.

2. Add the Parmesan cheese, and whisk until creamy and well blended.

3. Keep in a sealed glass container in the refrigerator for up to 1 week.

*STORAGE TIP* Mason jars are the perfect containers for keeping homemade salad dressings.

## VARIATIONS

There are many ways to make a Caesar dressing. Go ahead, be creative!

- Anchovy paste is a traditional addition to this dressing. Add 1 teaspoon to the recipe.
- ¼ cup of sour cream and minced garlic also adds a nice tang.

# AVOCADO-LIME CREMA

Think of this crema as a smoother guacamole that can also be used to top many different dishes. Try it on anything from salads to meaty entrées.

30-MINUTE
ONE POT
NO COOK
VEGETARIAN

**SERVES 4**
**PREP** 5 minutes

½ cup sour cream

½ avocado

1 garlic clove, finely minced

¼ cup fresh cilantro leaves

Juice of ½ lime

Pinch pink Himalayan salt

Pinch freshly ground black pepper

**Per Batch**
Calories: 346; Total Fat: 33g; Carbs: 14g; Net Carbs: 8g; Fiber: 6g; Protein: 4g

**Per Serving**
Calories: 87; Total Fat: 8g; Carbs: 4g; Net Carbs: 2g; Fiber: 2g; Protein: 1g

1. In a food processor (or blender), mix the sour cream, avocado, garlic, cilantro, lime juice, pink Himalayan salt, and pepper
until smooth and fully combined.

2. Spoon the sauce into an airtight glass jar and keep in the refrigerator for up to 3 days.

*INGREDIENT TIP* I like to put the crema in a zip-top bag and cut off a small corner for a piping bag. It looks beautiful piped over tacos, meat, deviled eggs, and more.

# CHUNKY BLUE CHEESE DRESSING

A great dressing for a wedge salad or a nice steak salad, but the dish I use it most often with is hot wings! There is nothing better than a crispy hot wing dipped in this cold-and-creamy blue cheese dressing.

30-MINUTE
ONE PAN
NO COOK

**SERVES 4**
**PREP** 5 minutes

½ cup sour cream

½ cup mayonnaise

Juice of ½ lemon

½ teaspoon
Worcestershire sauce

Pink Himalayan salt

Freshly ground
black pepper

2 ounces crumbled
blue cheese

**Per Batch**
Calories: 1225; Total Fat: 126g;
Carbs: 12g; Net Carbs: 11g;
Fiber: 1g; Protein: 18g

**Per Serving**
Calories: 306; Total Fat: 32g;
Carbs: 3g; Net Carbs: 3g;
Fiber: 0g; Protein: 7g

1. In a medium bowl, whisk the sour cream, mayonnaise, lemon juice, and Worcestershire sauce. Season with pink Himalayan salt and pepper, and whisk again until fully combined.

2. Fold in the crumbled blue cheese until well combined.

3. Keep in a sealed glass container in the refrigerator for up to 1 week.

*INGREDIENT TIP* You can adjust the amount of blue cheese crumbles to use in the dressing. I like it chunky.

# SRIRACHA MAYO

A sauce that makes any food better. Creamy and spicy, it is perfect for dipping chicken, veggies, and anything else you can grab.

**30-MINUTE**
**ONE PAN**
**NO COOK**
**VEGETARIAN**

**SERVES 4**
**PREP** 5 minutes

½ cup mayonnaise

2 tablespoons Sriracha sauce

½ teaspoon garlic powder

½ teaspoon onion powder

¼ teaspoon paprika

**Per Batch**
Calories: 804; Total Fat: 88g;
Carbs: 6g; Net Carbs: 5g;
Fiber: 1g; Protein: 2g

**Per Serving**
Calories: 201; Total Fat: 22g;
Carbs: 2g; Net Carbs: 1g;
Fiber: 0g; Protein: 1g

1. In a small bowl, whisk together the mayonnaise, Sriracha, garlic powder, onion powder, and paprika until well mixed.

2. Pour into an airtight glass container, and keep in the refrigerator for up to 1 week.

*INGREDIENT TIP* You can adjust the amount of Sriracha sauce to increase or decrease the spice level.

# AVOCADO MAYO

You can easily make your own mayonnaise using avocado. Maybe you're out of mayo, or maybe you just like making your own. Using avocado, you can make great mayo that is delicious mixed into dishes or used to top a keto-friendly burger or sandwich.

30-MINUTE
ONE PAN
NO COOK
VEGETARIAN

**SERVES 4**
**PREP** 5 minutes

1 medium avocado, cut into chunks

½ teaspoon ground cayenne pepper

Juice of ½ lime

2 tablespoons fresh cilantro leaves (optional)

Pinch pink Himalayan salt

¼ cup olive oil

**Per Batch**
Calories: 231; Total Fat: 20g;
Carbs: 16g; Net Carbs: 5g;
Fiber: 10g; Protein: 3g

**Per Serving**
Calories: 58; Total Fat: 5g;
Carbs: 4g; Net Carbs: 1g;
Fiber: 3g; Protein: 1g

1. In a food processor (or blender), blend the avocado, cayenne pepper, lime juice, cilantro, and pink Himalayan salt until all the ingredients are well combined and smooth.

2. Slowly incorporate the olive oil, adding 1 tablespoon at a time, pulsing the food processor in between.

3. Keep in a sealed glass container in the refrigerator for up to 1 week.

*INGREDIENT TIP* You want your avocado to be ripe: not too hard, but not too soft. When choosing at the market, a perfectly ripe avocado should just yield to light thumb pressure next to the stem. This trick doesn't bruise the avocado like other methods.

# PEANUT SAUCE

Peanut sauce will bring your chicken dishes to another level. I also like to toss zoodles with it, and I often just use it with any dish where I want to bring in some Asian flavor.

30-MINUTE
ONE PAN
NO COOK
VEGETARIAN

**SERVES 4**
**PREP** 5 minutes

½ cup creamy peanut butter
(I use Justin's)

2 tablespoons soy sauce
(or coconut aminos)

1 teaspoon Sriracha sauce

1 teaspoon toasted
sesame oil

1 teaspoon garlic powder

**Per Batch**
Calories: 741; Total Fat: 61g;
Carbs: 33g; Net Carbs: 25g;
Fiber: 8g; Protein: 27g

**Per Serving**
Calories: 185; Total Fat: 15g;
Carbs: 8g; Net Carbs: 6g;
Fiber: 2g; Protein: 7g

1.  In a food processor (or blender), blend the peanut butter, soy sauce, Sriracha sauce, sesame oil, and garlic powder until thoroughly mixed.

2.  Pour into an airtight glass container and keep in the refrigerator for up to 1 week.

*INGREDIENT TIP* For added texture, use chunky peanut butter.

# GARLIC AIOLI

Garlic aioli sauce always sounds so fancy when it is on a restaurant menu, but it really couldn't be easier to make. The chives and parsley are not mandatory, but I love the addition of fresh herbs in a sauce like this one.

30-MINUTE
ONE POT
NO COOK
VEGETARIAN

**SERVES 4**
**PREP** 5 minutes, plus
30 minutes to chill

½ cup mayonnaise

2 garlic cloves, minced

Juice of 1 lemon

1 tablespoon chopped
fresh flat-leaf Italian parsley

1 teaspoon chopped chives

Pink Himalayan salt

Freshly ground
black pepper

**Per Batch**
Calories: 817; Total Fat: 88g;
Carbs: 11g; Net Carbs: 9g;
Fiber: 2g; Protein: 2g

**Per Serving**
Calories: 204; Total Fat: 22g;
Carbs: 3g; Net Carbs: 2g;
Fiber: 1g; Protein: 1g

1. In a food processor (or blender), combine the mayonnaise, garlic, lemon juice, parsley, and chives, and season with pink Himalayan salt and pepper. Blend until fully combined.

2. Pour into a sealed glass container and chill in the refrigerator for at least 30 minutes before serving. (This sauce will keep in the fridge for up to 1 week.)

*INGREDIENT TIP* Mince the garlic as finely as possible for best results. You can even grate it with a zester if you have one.

# TZATZIKI

Tzatziki sauce is so delicious. I love going to the Mediterranean bistro by my house for a meal. They have tzatziki, and I always ask for extra. One day I finally made it myself. The key is getting all the water out of the cucumber. That aside, tzatziki is super easy to make.

NO COOK
VEGETARIAN

**SERVES 4**
**PREP** 10 minutes,
plus at least 30 minutes
to chill

½ large English cucumber,
unpeeled

1½ cups Greek yogurt
(I use Fage)

2 tablespoons olive oil

Large pinch pink
Himalayan salt

Large pinch freshly ground
black pepper

Juice of ½ lemon

2 garlic cloves,
finely minced

1 tablespoon fresh dill

**Per Batch**
Calories: 596; Total Fat: 44g;
Carbs: 20g; Net Carbs: 18g;
Fiber: 2g; Protein: 32g

**Per Serving**
Calories: 149; Total Fat: 11g;
Carbs: 5g; Net Carbs: 5g;
Fiber: 1g; Protein: 8g

1. Halve the cucumber lengthwise, and use a spoon to scoop out and discard the seeds.

2. Grate the cucumber with a zester or grater onto a large plate lined with a few layers of paper towels. Close the paper towels around the grated cucumber, and squeeze as much water out of it as you can. (This can take a while and can require multiple paper towels. You can also allow it to drain overnight in a strainer or wrapped in a few layers of cheesecloth in the fridge if you have the time.)

3. In a food processor (or blender), blend the yogurt, olive oil, pink Himalayan salt, pepper, lemon juice, and garlic until fully combined.

4. Transfer the mixture to a medium bowl, and mix in the fresh dill and grated cucumber.

5. I like to chill this sauce for at least 30 minutes before serving. Keep in a sealed glass container in the refrigerator for up to 1 week.

*INGREDIENT TIP* Mince the garlic cloves as finely as possible for best results. You can use sour cream instead of Greek yogurt.

# ALFREDO SAUCE

There is nothing like a warm bowl of fettuccine Alfredo with its rich, buttery, creamy sauce. In the winter, I love to use Miracle Noodles of the fettuccine variety and top them with this sauce, served with some grilled chicken cooked with fresh herbs. The delicious ingredients are always in my kitchen, so it is simple to pull the sauce together.

30-MINUTE
ONE POT
VEGETARIAN

**SERVES 2**
**PREP** 5 minutes
**COOK** 10 minutes

4 tablespoons butter

2 ounces cream cheese

1 cup heavy
(whipping) cream

½ cup grated
Parmesan cheese

1 garlic clove, finely minced

1 teaspoon dried Italian
seasoning

Pink Himalayan salt

Freshly ground
black pepper

**Per Batch**
Calories: 1175; Total Fat: 120g;
Carbs: 8g; Net Carbs: 8g;
Fiber: 0g; Protein: 21g

**Per Serving**
Calories: 294; Total Fat: 30g;
Carbs: 2g; Net Carbs: 2g;
Fiber: 0g; Protein: 5g

1. In a heavy medium saucepan over medium heat, combine the butter, cream cheese, and heavy cream. Whisk slowly and constantly until the butter and cream cheese melt.

2. Add the Parmesan, garlic, and Italian seasoning. Continue to whisk until everything is well blended. Turn the heat to medium-low and simmer, stirring occasionally, for 5 to 8 minutes to allow the sauce to blend and thicken.

3. Season with pink Himalayan salt and pepper, and stir to combine.

4. Toss with your favorite hot, precooked, keto-friendly noodles and serve.

5. Keep this sauce in a sealed glass container in the refrigerator for up to 4 days.

*INGREDIENT TIP* You can also use a delicious grated cheese that combines Parmesan, Asiago, and Romano.

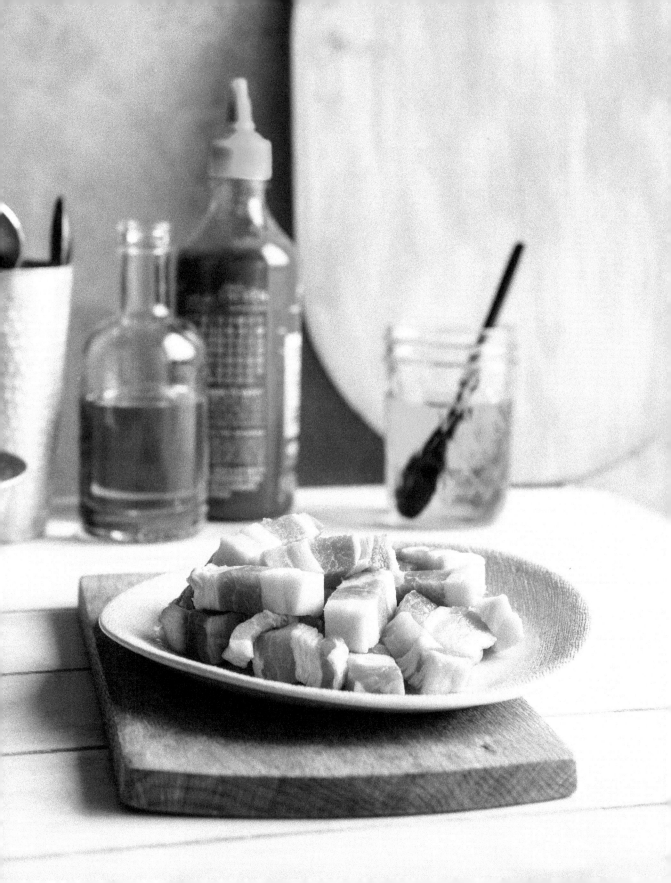

# THE DIRTY DOZEN™ & THE CLEAN FIFTEEN™

A nonprofit environmental watchdog organization called Environmental Working Group (EWG) looks at data supplied by the US Department of Agriculture (USDA) and the Food and Drug Administration (FDA) about pesticide residues. Each year it compiles a list of the best and worst pesticide loads found in commercial crops. You can use these lists to decide which fruits and vegetables to buy organic to minimize your exposure to pesticides and which produce is considered safe enough to buy conventionally. This does not mean they are pesticide-free, though, so wash these fruits and vegetables thoroughly.

These lists change every year, so make sure you look up the most recent one before you fill your shopping cart. You'll find the most recent lists, as well as a guide to pesticides in produce, at EWG.org/FoodNews.

## DIRTY DOZEN

| | | |
|---|---|---|
| Apples | Nectarines | *In addition to the Dirty Dozen, the EWG added two types of produce contaminated with highly toxic organophosphate insecticides:* |
| Celery | Peaches | |
| Cherries | Spinach | |
| Cherry tomatoes | Strawberries | |
| Cucumbers | Sweet bell peppers | Kale/Collard greens |
| Grapes | Tomatoes | Hot peppers |

## CLEAN FIFTEEN

| | | |
|---|---|---|
| Asparagus | Eggplant | Onions |
| Avocados | Grapefruit | Papayas |
| Cabbage | Honeydew melon | Pineapples |
| Cantaloupe | Kiwifruits | Sweet corn |
| Cauliflower | Mangos | Sweet peas (frozen) |

# APPENDIX B
# MEASUREMENT CONVERSIONS

## OVEN TEMPERATURES

| FAHRENHEIT | CELSIUS (APPROXIMATE) |
|---|---|
| 250°F | 120°C |
| 300°F | 150°C |
| 325°F | 165°C |
| 350°F | 180°C |
| 375°F | 190°C |
| 400°F | 200°C |
| 425°F | 220°C |
| 450°F | 230°C |

## WEIGHT EQUIVALENTS

| US STANDARD | METRIC (APPROXIMATE) |
|---|---|
| ½ ounce | 15 g |
| 1 ounce | 30 g |
| 2 ounces | 60 g |
| 4 ounces | 115 g |
| 8 ounces | 225 g |
| 12 ounces | 340 g |
| 16 ounces or 1 pound | 455 g |

## VOLUME EQUIVALENTS (LIQUID)

| US STANDARD | US STANDARD (OUNCES) | METRIC (APPROXIMATE) |
|---|---|---|
| 2 tablespoons | 1 fl. oz. | 30 mL |
| ¼ cup | 2 fl. oz. | 60 mL |
| ½ cup | 4 fl. oz. | 120 mL |
| 1 cup | 8 fl. oz. | 240 mL |
| 1½ cups | 12 fl. oz. | 355 mL |
| 2 cups or 1 pint | 16 fl. oz. | 475 mL |
| 4 cups or 1 quart | 32 fl. oz. | 1 L |
| 1 gallon | 128 fl. oz. | 4 L |

## VOLUME EQUIVALENTS (DRY)

| US STANDARD | METRIC (APPROXIMATE) |
|---|---|
| ⅛ teaspoon | 0.5 mL |
| ¼ teaspoon | 1 mL |
| ½ teaspoon | 2 mL |
| ¾ teaspoon | 4 mL |
| 1 teaspoon | 5 mL |
| 1 tablespoon | 15 mL |
| ¼ cup | 59 mL |
| ⅓ cup | 79 mL |
| ½ cup | 118 mL |
| ⅔ cup | 156 mL |
| ¾ cup | 177 mL |
| 1 cup | 235 mL |
| 2 cups or 1 pint | 475 mL |
| 3 cups | 700 mL |
| 4 cups or 1 quart | 1 L |

# REFERENCES

Centers for Disease Control and Prevention, National Center for Health Statistics. "Dietary Intake for Adults Aged 20 and Over." 2016. www.cdc.gov/nchs/fastats/diet.htm.

Wilson, Jacob, and Ryan Lowery. *The Ketogenic Bible: The Authoritative Guide to Ketosis*. Victory Belt Publishing, 2017. This book is an excellent resource for a deep dive into the science of keto and ketosis.

# RESOURCES

### KETOINTHECITY.COM
On my blog I feature Keto FAQs, interviews, and many recipes.

### RULED ME (RULED.ME)
This is the macro calculator that I use and link on my blog.

### CARB MANAGER APP (CARBMANAGER.COM)
This app is my favorite for tracking my food and macros.

There are many great keto-friendly brands, but sometimes they are difficult to find at a typical grocery store. I've listed some of my favorite products below, and provided my discount codes to save you some money on your purchases.

### KNOW FOODS
10% off
knowfoods.com
Code: KETOINTHECITY

### KETO FRIDGE
10% off
ketofridge.com
Code: KETOINTHECITY

### LEGENDARY FOODS
10% off
legendaryfoodsonline.com
Code: KETOINTHECITY

### PERFECT KETO
10% off
perfectketo.com
Code: KETOINTHECITY

### CHOC ZERO
10% off
choczero.com
Code: KETOINTHECITY

### EQUIP FOODS
10% off
equipfoods.com
Code: KETOINTHECITY

### KETO KOOKIE
10% off
ketokookie.com
Code: KETOINTHECITY

### MIRACLE NOODLE
10% off
miraclenoodle.com
Code: KETOINTHECITY

### KETTLE & FIRE BONE BROTH
15% off
kettleandfire.com
Code: KETOINTHECITY 15

# RECIPE TITLE INDEX

# RECIPE TYPE INDEX

# INDEX

Cream
 Alfredo Sauce, 175
 Bacon Cheeseburger Casserole, 135–136
 Bacon, Spinach, and Avocado Egg Wrap, 28
 Blueberry-Blackberry Ice Pops, 141
 Blue Cheese Pork Chops, 122
 Broccoli-Cheese Soup, 44
 Cheesy Cauliflower Soup, 45
 Chocolate Mousse, 157
 Coffee Ice Pops, 143
 Cream Cheese Muffins, 39
 Creamy Tomato-Basil Soup, 43
 Dark-Chocolate Strawberry Bark, 161
 Double-Pork Frittata, 23
 "Frosty" Chocolate Shake, 148
 Fudge Ice Pops, 144
 Mint–Chocolate Chip Ice Cream, 158–159
 Orange Cream Float, 146
 Root Beer Float, 145
 Scallops with Creamy Bacon Sauce, 93
 Spicy Breakfast Scramble, 25
 Strawberry Cheesecake Mousse, 149
 Strawberry-Lime Ice Pops, 142
 Strawberry Shake, 147
Cream cheese
 Alfredo Sauce, 175
 Bacon-Jalapeño Egg Cups, 26
 Bacon-Wrapped Jalapeños, 86
 Berry Cheesecake Fat Bomb, 151
 Buffalo Chicken Dip, 82
 Cheesy Bacon and Broccoli Chicken, 107
 Cheesy Cauliflower Soup, 45
 Chocolate-Avocado Pudding, 160
 Chocolate Mousse, 157
 Cream Cheese and Coconut Flour Pancakes
  or Waffles, 35–36
 Cream Cheese Muffins, 39
 Creamy Tomato-Basil Soup, 43
 Crustless Cheesecake Bites, 153
 Lemonade Fat Bomb, 150
 Pancake "Cake," 37
 Pumpkin Crustless Cheesecake
  Bites, 154
 Salami, Pepperoncini, and Cream Cheese
  Pinwheels, 84

 Smoked Salmon and Cream Cheese
  Roll-Ups, 29
 Strawberry Cheesecake Mousse, 149
 Strawberry Shake, 147
 Taco Soup, 46
Cucumbers
 Chicken-Pecan Salad Cucumber Bites, 81
 Mediterranean Cucumber Salad, 53
 Seared-Salmon Shirataki Rice Bowls, 97–98
 Steak and Egg Bibimbap, 130–131
 Tomato, Avocado, and Cucumber Salad, 73
 Tzatziki, 174

## D

Dairy products, 5. *See also specific*
 to avoid, 9
 to enjoy, 8
Dill
 Creamy Dill Salmon, 100
 Double-Pork Frittata, 23
 Tzatziki, 174
Dining out, 6, 41
Dressings
 Caesar Dressing, 167
 Chunky Blue Cheese Dressing, 169
 Dijon Vinaigrette, 165
 Green Goddess Dressing, 166

## E

Eggs
 Avocado Egg Salad Lettuce Cups, 54
 Bacon and Egg Cauliflower Hash, 27
 Bacon Cheeseburger Casserole,
  135–136
 Bacon-Jalapeño Egg Cups, 26
 Bacon, Spinach, and Avocado Egg
  Wrap, 28
 BLT Breakfast Salad, 31
 Breakfast Quesadilla, 38
 Cheesy Egg and Spinach Nest, 32
 Cream Cheese and Coconut Flour Pancakes
  or Waffles, 35–36
 Cream Cheese Muffins, 39

# ACKNOWLEDGMENTS

TO MY PARENTS  I love you and thank you for always allowing me to believe that I could truly do anything if I worked hard enough.

TO KAIA  Having you as my daughter is my greatest joy. I love you to the moon and back, and I am so happy to always have you by my side.

TO MY FRIENDS AND FAMILY  I am so inspired by my tribe and I am so grateful to have such an amazing group of people around me. You are the people you surround yourself with, and I am lucky to be surrounded by greatness.

TO THE KETO COMMUNITY  I am so grateful to have found the passionate and supportive keto community on Instagram and online. You are an incredible group of people, each fighting different challenges but all trying to better yourselves. You all inspire me, and I hope I have been able to inspire you in return.

## ABOUT THE AUTHOR

JEN FISCH, creator of the blog *Keto In The City*, is passionate about offering simple solutions for following the ketogenic lifestyle. She is a single, working mother who has battled autoimmune disorders for 20 years and has turned to the kitchen to find simple, delicious ways to make the ketogenic diet work for her busy lifestyle.

With a loyal Instagram following at her page @ketointhecity_, her growing YouTube channel *Keto In The City*, and more than 100,000 visitors to her blog KetoInTheCity.com, Jen is one of the top influencers in the ketogenic space.

She is not a nutritionist or trained chef, just a determined mom who searched high and low for a way of eating that would reduce the inflammation caused by her autoimmune disorders and allow her to feel like the very best version of herself. She lives with her daughter in Hermosa Beach, California.

CPSIA information can be obtained
at www.ICGtesting.com
Printed in the USA
BVHW051711190421
605119BV00003B/4